rest + calm

GREEN TREE
Bloomsbury Publishing Plc
50 Bedford Square, London, WC1B 3DP, UK
29 Earlsfort Terrace, Dublin 2, Ireland

BLOOMSBURY, GREEN TREE and the Green Tree logo are trademarks of Bloomsbury Publishing Plc

First published in Great Britain 2022

© Paula Hines, 2022
Instagram: @ucanyoga1 / Website: ucanyoga.co.uk

Illustrations © Chloe Smart, 2022
Instagram: @chloesmartprint / Website: chloesmartprint.com

Paula Hines has asserted her right under the Copyright, Designs and Patents Act, 1988,
to be identified as Author of this work

A catalogue record for this book is available from the British Library

Library of Congress Cataloguing-in-Publication data has been applied for

ISBN: PB: 978-1-4729-9369-4; eBook: 978-1-4729-9368-7; ePdf: 978-1-4729-9367-0

2 4 6 8 10 9 7 5 3 1

Typeset in Agenda
Designed by Austin Taylor

Printed and bound in China by Toppan Leefung Printing

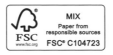

To find out more about our authors and books visit www.bloomsbury.com
and sign up for our newsletters

rest + calm

Gentle yoga and mindful practices
to nurture and restore yourself

PAULA HINES

GREEN TREE
LONDON • OXFORD • NEW YORK • NEW DELHI • SYDNEY

*For Mum, my brother and
my grandmothers.*

CONTENTS

FOREWORD by Bo Forbes

I first met Paula Hines in 2017, while teaching a workshop in London. We had the chance to enjoy several conversations throughout the three-day weekend; I was struck by her vibrant dedication to the therapeutic applications of yoga for physical, emotional and social well-being. In the years since, I have had more opportunities to learn with Paula and to appreciate her contributions to the field of yoga.

A hallmark of Paula's body of work is its indivisibility from who she is personally and from the issues that matter to her, such as women's health and social justice. In an age where it is perhaps easy to be buffeted about by the interests of the moment, Paula has shown a steady allegiance to the dissemination of yoga's deeper teachings. And despite the myriad pressures that modern Western yoga instructors face to teach physically challenging forms of yoga, Paula concentrates her energy on practices imbued with rest, self-care and restoration.

Paula has steeped in the traditions of yoga and mindfulness in a deep and meaningful way. Her other offerings are outgrowths of this: her passion for writing and regular column (Teacher's Tales) in *Om Yoga & Lifestyle Magazine*. Her weekly 'Switch Off Sundays' that encourage people to unplug from social media. Her workshops on menopause and perimenopause. Her communications on social justice.

Rest + Calm is a beautiful book, an extension of Paula's direct experience with contemplative practice in a rapidly changing world. Her 365 Savasana Project bears testimony to the fact that she has earned her teaching credibility through personal suffering, thoughtful reflection and breakthroughs. She has committed to the practices in this book in an ongoing and meaningful way. She has reflected upon them in her own svadhyaya (self-study). And she has adapted them for multiple needs and real-life demands so she can offer them to others. Paula is not simply a good writer; her experience weaves a tangible web of safety around the reader, a holding environment for growth and transformation.

Paula artfully integrates important background and context with key elements of yoga philosophy, such as the eight limbs of yoga and the koshas. She weaves in mindfulness philosophy and practices such as loving kindness meditation. She offers therapeutic sequences for a number of conditions and experiences, from insomnia and anxiety to grief and exhaustion and parenting – all in a down-to-earth, accessible way.

Part I of the book, 'Rest', contains restorative yoga postures along with a gentle progressive relaxation that serves as a prelude. Part 2 of the book, 'Calm', offers an intricate and comprehensive section of pranayama and key additional practices: mudras, yoga nidra (yogic sleep), a body scan and a wonderful section on creating strong boundaries.

As the SARS-CoV-2 pandemic has shown, the modern Western way of life is unsustainable. Anxiety, depression and PTSD are becoming pandemics of their own. We are in the midst of a global racial reckoning. Climate crisis and its resulting inequities are upon us. Authoritarianism is rising in multiple democratic countries.

The forces of dominant culture – white supremacy, patriarchy and capitalism – exert on us a pressure to move faster, produce better, demand more from ourselves and others. As Paula poignantly shares, neither yoga teachers nor practitioners are immune to these forces. This gem of a book is a guide to powerful practices for rest, reflection, self-care and the tending of community. The insight it contains is not a luxury, but a physical, emotional and spiritual imperative.

Bo Forbes, Psy.D., E-RYT, C-IAYT
Boston, Massachusetts
September, 2021

INTRODUCTION

You deserve rest even when – especially when – it feels like you have no time for it. And even when it feels like you have no time there are still ways to invite some calm into your day and improve your well-being.

You've probably heard the phrase 'You can't pour from an empty cup'. That's true. It's hard to be at your best and give your best if you're not rested. If productivity is your goal, then yes, rest will help you to be more productive and efficient. But the purpose of rest is not to be more productive.

So often our value is tied to our productivity, but you are worthy regardless of how productive you are. Rest is essential, not just for our individual selves, but also for each other – for our collective well-being. When we are not rested it is so much easier to go on autopilot and 'sleepwalk' through life.

You deserve rest simply because you were born. Yes, you. Really.

Hands up if you have been socialised to believe that resting is lazy or only for when you have completed everything on your to-do list (newsflash: the to-do list never *really* gets completed).

If you grew up in a capitalist society, the answer is likely to be yes. Or maybe you grew up in a home environment where the concept of rest didn't exist. Some of us had childhoods where we did not see our elders rest or, if we appeared to be doing nothing, we were soon given a chore to fill that space.

Rest is good for you

Yes, rest is good for you, but beyond sleep (which itself is not always restful), how many of us allow ourselves time to properly rest?

It's common to feel that we simply don't have the time to rest. When we have so much to do, does it even matter? Surely you can just plough on and hope that things eventually slow down?

Possibly.

According to a study involving 18,000 people from 134 countries, people who had fewer hours of rest scored lower on a well-being scale.

What constitutes rest will not be the same for all of us. For a small percentage of people in this study, tiring out the body through vigorous exercise allowed the mind (if not the body) to rest. For the majority, though, time alone was what they craved, with 68 per cent of people saying they would like more rest. The most highly rated restful activities were often done alone, including reading, being in nature and doing nothing in particular.

Restorative yoga, which features in this book, could be described as looking like 'nothing in particular' – in the past I have joked that it can look like adult naptime. However, even though it might appear as though nothing is happening, there is deep rejuvenation taking place beneath the surface in a way that zoning out in front of the TV watching back-to-back box sets does not achieve.

Yet it seems that resting causes some people to worry about the things they aren't, or feel they should be, doing. In the same study, it was noted that when asked which words they most associated with rest, almost 9 per cent of people chose the words 'guilty' or 'stress-inducing'. However, carrying on regardless is not a viable long-term option. Even the most resilient person deprived of proper rest will break eventually.

In this book I invite you to give yourself permission to rest. And if you feel that's not something you can do, then I am officially giving you that permission right now.

How to use this book

This is not a book that requires you to read it from cover to cover. Think of Rest + Calm as a rest toolkit, which you can dip into whenever you need to.

The first part of this book, REST, focuses on the nourishing practice of restorative yoga and guides you through various poses and sequences. If restorative yoga is totally new to you, then I would suggest reading the Why restorative yoga? section which will provide you with an overview and the Beginning your restorative practice section for tips that will help you get the best out of your practice before you delve into the poses and sequences.

The second part of this book, CALM, offers practical tips and techniques beyond the yoga poses for intentional day-to-day living and emotional rescue for those moments when it feels as though you have no time.

While much of what I present in this book appears relatively simple, it's not always easy, not least because it requires you to give back to yourself. Learning to rest – to let go of the lure of constant busyness – does take practice. But this is not about perfection. All that is required is a willingness to try and to know that prioritising yourself in this way is far from selfish. When you're rested, it's good for everyone around you. Imagine how different the world would be if we were all well-rested.

Why does rest matter so much to me and why do I care about you being rested?

My story: The yoga teacher who was tired and wired

I came into teaching yoga off the back of a 14-year career working full-time in television and 10 years as a yoga practitioner. In fact, it was back pain from too many hours sitting and stress from work that led me to yoga in the first place. What kept me coming back was the effect yoga had on me. As much as I loved my TV job, I knew I had reached a turning point. When the possibility of redundancy was on the horizon, it was the catalyst for me to take the leap.

It was exciting (and somewhat scary) to start from scratch in my thirties – to embark on yoga teacher training, meet new people and then to begin teaching. I had a very slow start, setting up my own drop-in weekly class locally, often to find that no one would show up, but then the pace picked up to what at times seemed like lightning speed.

Two years into teaching full-time I was travelling all over London teaching multiple classes weekly to groups, to corporate clients in the City, to private clients in their homes. I was regularly teaching on yoga retreats and even assisting, then becoming a tutor on a well-respected yoga teacher training course.

I was incredibly fortunate with the opportunities that came my way, but while there were lots of ups, there were plenty of downs too. As with many things, outsiders tend only to see what appear to be the shiny successes and not the obstacles, the disappointments and the failures. I found I was working a lot in order to scrape by financially. This also meant that out of necessity I often worked when I was unwell. (These are realities for so many of us in all walks of life.) Plus the people pleaser in me (now happily in recovery!) never wanted to let other people down.

The very nature of teaching, especially full-time, means you're often giving a lot. The trouble was, I was in survival mode, working so much, saying yes to everything for fear that if I said no the opportunity would not come back around again. The result? Caring for myself slipped further and further down my list of day-to-day priorities.

This was alongside health issues and challenges in my personal life. I experienced sudden hair loss, which a doctor advised me was connected to the stress I was under and then my father passed away. Being self-employed and feeling unable to take the time to grieve, I continued to work.

One of the cherished things in my routine that I had managed to hold on to as a non-negotiable was a weekly Sunday morning run with a friend. One Sunday, as we ended our run with our usual sit-down in a café, out of nowhere I burst into tears. I tried to play it down by joking that I was just tired and emotional. Those tears in front of my friend were a turning point and I knew something had to change. 'You need a holiday,' was my friend's advice as she lent a supportive ear.

I knew that a holiday anytime soon was not possible, but when I got home I did what I could in that moment – I lay down on the floor for 20 minutes. As I lay there, covered in a blanket with soft support under my head and knees, I felt the physical tension release from my body. Something profound happened during that 20 minutes. My perspective shifted. My immediate thought was, 'I should do this more.'

A common pitfall for newer teachers when moving from being a student of yoga to teaching full-time is that their own yoga practice falters. I had fallen into this trap.

I first started practising restorative yoga when I was still working in television, then later, when as a brand-new teacher injury reared its head, I turned towards restorative yoga and away from the more intensive, dynamic and physical practices that I realised were leaving me in pain.

This is when I deeply understood the therapeutic benefits of restorative yoga. I knew that I wanted to study this practice and to be able to share it with others. However, along the way with life, transitioning from being an employee to self-employed and what felt like constant busyness, I had forgotten the words of Judith Hanson Lasater:

'[Restorative yoga] is magic and the magic is that it doesn't work if you don't do it.'

Emerging from that 20-minute savasana on that Sunday afternoon, I knew I needed to make different choices.

The power of rest

I had completed my restorative yoga teacher training with the renowned teacher Judith Hanson Lasater a couple of years prior to that day when I broke down in front of my friend. I was particularly interested in studying with Judith not only because of her decades of experience, but also because her teacher was the person who is known for developing the practice of restorative yoga – B.K.S. Iyengar. Judith told us that restorative yoga is a practice that yoga teachers need to do. I didn't understand that at the time, but by this point it made complete sense.

In yoga, savasana – the pose that usually comes at the end of a class – is described as the easiest pose to do, yet the hardest to master. It requires the willingness to be still. I decided to practise a restorative savasana (the foundation pose of restorative yoga, which you will learn in this book) for 20 minutes a day, every day for a year. I stayed true to this and whatever was happening, even when I was travelling for work, I found 20 minutes daily to practise. The result was transformative.

While the things in my life did not necessarily change, how I faced and dealt with them did. This is not to say that you have to do exactly what I did, but the point is that there is real power in a consistent rest practice, far beyond the idea of being more productive or getting more sleep. In fact, restorative yoga can help to improve sleep, but, more importantly, restorative yoga can help us face ourselves with compassion.

part 1

rest

Why restorative yoga?

The clue is in the name – RESTorative yoga is excellent for facilitating proper rest and relaxation in both body and mind. Restorative yoga is a receptive, soothing practice where you are supported and held – how many of us could deeply benefit from more of that?

Many of the restorative poses we know were developed by B.K.S. Iyengar of Pune, India, or inspired by his therapeutic work. Well-known for his use of props, Mr Iyengar experimented with them, modifying poses until his students could practice without strain, and he also explored how these versions of the poses could help people recover from injury or illness.

The reason why props are important is because they provide support for our physical body and enhance comfort. The more comfortable you are, the more the body is able to drop into a state of relaxation and rest. But it need not be complicated – far from it. Though you certainly could invest in special yoga props if you wanted to, you don't have to. Your prop could be as simple as a wall or sofa in your home. Other examples of items from around your home that you can use as props for restorative yoga include, but are not limited to:

- Bed pillows
- Cushions
- Blankets
- Throws from your sofa or bed
- Towels
- Soft scarves
- Eye pillows or eye masks
- Belts
- Your bed

The list goes on, but we'll get more into props and how you can use them later.

The stress connection

In our modern-day existence (and certainly since 2020 and the impact of Covid-19), more and more of us are increasingly living in a heightened, chronically stressed state. Depending on our lived experience, some of us have been in this state for a long time. In other words, we are often in a sympathetic nervous system state. The sympathetic nervous system (SNS) is the part of our autonomic nervous system that switches on what is called our fight/flight/freeze response. For our ancient ancestors this would have been caused by an immediate threat, like fleeing a predator intent on eating them for dinner. In these situations, the heart rate, muscle tension and blood pressure would increase as they prepared to escape, while all the systems not needed in that moment, like digestion, were shut down.

Once they escaped the threat of being an animal's next meal, their adrenals would stop pumping stress hormones through their bodies and everything would re-set. But now, threats – from the point of our nervous system – are more likely to take the form of things like health issues, racial discrimination, financial worries, job insecurity, relationship concerns and so much more. On top of this, add living busy lives with near-constant overstimulation from our surroundings (never mind our smartphones) and is it any wonder many of us feel frazzled?

These modern-day 'threats' don't disappear so easily. The result? Our adrenals continue to produce stress hormones and we stay in that SNS state. The SNS does a good job of fulfilling its role to save our lives, when we are in danger, but the trouble is that nowadays, because the SNS is so over-stimulated, most of us are running on the SNS constantly. This is where stress becomes chronic. That prolonged stress can be harmful and may even eventually manifest as illness.

Enter restorative yoga

This is where restorative yoga comes in and where it can be helpful. Research has shown that restorative yoga can activate the parasympathetic nervous system (PNS) – the part of our autonomic nervous system responsible for our rest/digest/tend/restore activities. So restorative yoga can be especially beneficial when we are experiencing chronic stress and we feel tired all the time.

The relaxation response

The 'relaxation response' is a term widely popularised by cardiologist and professor Dr Herbert Benson in his 1975 book of the same name. It is the opposite to fight/flight (the body's stress response). Over 45 years ago Dr Benson outlined the benefits of 10 to 20 minutes a day of practice to

THE VAGUS NERVE

The vagus nerve is the longest of the cranial nerves. 'Vagus' is Latin for 'wandering', so it's aptly named, because the vagus nerve travels from the brain stem down the front of the body, meandering from the facial muscles, throat and inner ear to the lungs, diaphragm, stomach and intestines. Stimulating this nerve activates a relaxation response of the parasympathetic nervous system. Therefore, practices such as restorative yoga, pranayama (breathing practices, including diaphragmatic breathing – see the CALM section) and meditation (including loving kindness – see the CALM section) have been shown to be effective for stimulating or toning the vagus nerve.

counteract the stress response. Restorative yoga is one of a number of ways to achieve this, as the very nature of the practice facilitates deep relaxation. A very important aspect of restorative yoga (and also where it differs from other forms of yoga) is that it gives our bodies the opportunity to truly rest and, for our health and well-being, rest is a necessity rather than a luxury. As restorative yoga is particularly effective in addressing chronic stress, any of the practices in this book will be helpful if stress management is an objective for you. Aside from easing stress, just a few of the reported benefits of restorative yoga include:

- Nervous system regulation
- Boosts the immune system
- Improves energy levels
- Eases anxiety and depression
- Improves sleep
- Eases muscular tension
- Reduces blood pressure
- Balances hormones
- Aids recovery from injury and illness

This is not to say that restorative yoga (or yoga in general) is a cure-all, but it can certainly be one of the things in your toolkit. Don't be surprised if, with practice, your experience shifts, clarity comes to you and solutions arise to problems that you had not been able to resolve beforehand. This is a simple yet profound practice, so if you allow it to, it can change your perspective for the better, as well as providing deep renewal.

You can certainly feel better by spending a few minutes in one pose every so often, though to reap deep benefits a degree of consistency – practice – is required. Like so many things that do us good, we need to actually 'do' the thing not just once, but on a regular basis. By doing a little on a regular basis, you may surprise yourself by finding that your relationship with rest improves in ways you never imagined possible. Modern life can make us disconnect from our bodies, from ourselves. Restorative yoga is a practice that can welcome us back home to ourselves.

Beginning your restorative practice

For each practice I will offer prop suggestions. However, please feel free to be creative with what you have around your home to ensure you feel as comfortable as possible and have the support you need. For instance, I sometimes use the seat cushions from my sofa instead of bed pillows.

Be comfortable

'*Sthira sukham asanam*' – sutra 2.46

The most common translation of this sutra from Patanjali's *Yoga Sutras*, one of the key yoga texts, is '*asana (posture) should be stable or steady (sthira) and comfortable (sukha).*' There is a part of you that is always steady and always at ease. The practice of yoga can help us to access and reside in that place. In terms of your restorative yoga practice, the more comfortable you are in your poses, the easier you will find it to simply be.

When you're comfortable, it becomes easier for the body (and mind) to drop into a relaxed state. If you are distracted by something – for example, you feel as though you need another cushion under your head – then you won't be comfortable and therefore you will not be able to relax.

When you get into your pose, take a few moments to note how you feel. A good question to ask yourself is whether there is anything you can do to make yourself even 10 per cent more comfortable. Also, consider how you might feel in the pose two to five minutes in. Adjust and re-adjust as much as you need to until you reach a point where you feel so comfortable that you no longer have a desire to move. Taking your time with this step will pay dividends while you are in your restorative pose.

It's practice not perfect – be kind yourself

You can choose to stay in a number of the poses in this book for up to 20 minutes at a time, but if two to three minutes is all you have that is absolutely OK. It's only natural that some days you will have more time than others. One of my mottos for practising which you might find helpful is, 'Some is better than none'. Please don't feel that your practice must look and be the same every time you do it. This is absolutely not about perfection.

There are eight limbs of yoga (see box opposite), of which the poses are only one. As you can see, the poses (asana) are in fact the third limb. The first limb is the yamas (known as moral ethics or ways of 'right living') and the first of the yamas is ahimsa, a Sanskrit word that translates as 'non-violence' or 'non-harming'. Ahimsa includes how we treat ourselves, as well how we treat as others and our environment. I mention this here, because so often we are our own toughest critics. Think of all the times in your life when you have judged yourself far more harshly than you would someone else. So please be kind to yourself in your approach to your practice.

Bed or floor?

While you can practise most of the postures in this book lying on a bed (which can also be an option if getting up and down off the floor is a challenge), you might want to avoid this if you don't want to risk falling asleep. To practise lying on the floor, I would suggest you place a blanket or throw on the ground to lie on. If your floor is not carpeted, I would definitely recommend this. If you do have a yoga mat or similar, then you can absolutely use that and you can certainly place a comfy blanket on top of your mat too for extra cosiness.

THE EIGHT LIMBS OF YOGA

The name 'eight limbs' stems from the Sanskrit term 'ashtanga'. These guidelines on living a life of purpose and meaning are outlined in the *Yoga Sutras of Patanjali*:

1 **Yamas:** the five moral ethics

- Ahimsa (non-violence)
- Satya (truthfulness)
- Asteya (non-stealing)
- Brahmacharya (moderation)
- Aparigraha (non-attachment)

2 **Niyamas:** the five observances

- Saucha (cleanliness)
- Santosha (contentment)
- Tapas (discipline, burning determination or enthusiasm)
- Svadhyaya (self-study)
- Ishvara pranidhana (surrender, devotion)

3 **Asana:** postures
4 **Pranayama:** life force expansion, mindful breathing
5 **Pratyahara:** withdrawal of the senses
6 **Dharana:** concentration
7 **Dhyana:** meditation
8 **Samadhi:** pure bliss, oneness

A dedicated spot

You might wish to have a specific place where you practise – maybe in a particular room. For instance, for me this is usually on the floor next to my sofa at home – this also makes it easy to use my sofa as a prop if I want to. Likewise, I know some people like to practise on the floor next to their bed, which allows the option of using their bed as a prop. Having a dedicated spot that you associate with your rest practice could also be one way of helping to develop consistency and allow this to become a positive ritual.

Stay warm

Even if you feel warm or very hot before you practise, it's a good idea to have a blanket (or similar) to hand that you can use to cover your body with once you're ready to settle into your restorative pose. This is because it's common (and normal) for the body temperature to begin to drop once we are still for a while. (Think of how we cover ourselves with duvets, sheets or blankets to go to sleep at bedtime.) It is better to have a blanket easily within reach and not need to use it than to be all settled and comfy, only to then get cold and fidgety and have to get up or curtail your time in a pose that you were enjoying. Related to this, you might want to have socks handy too!

Block out the light

Just as important as having a blanket to hand, having something to cover your eyes can also enhance your practice. Light is a powerful stimulant to the brain and can be a barrier to being able to relax fully. If you prefer the lights to be out when you go to sleep at night, then having an eye cover is a good idea. A sleep mask or eye pillow can be ideal, but just as effective is a soft scarf to place over your eyes.

That said, if the idea of covering or indeed closing your eyes is not at all comfortable or safe for you, then if it's possible to reduce the light coming into the space where you intend to practise by drawing the curtains or blinds, please do this.

Alternatively, if you would prefer to keep your eyes open, then practise softening your gaze to a single spot in your eyeline so that the muscles around your eyes can be relaxed. There may be a natural tendency for the eyes to dart around, especially if the mind is busy, but the act of softening the gaze in one place will be more calming for your nervous system and will therefore help to facilitate relaxation. If you find your gaze drifting off, then each time this happens gently guide your gaze back to that single spot.

Using a timer

A timer can be helpful so that you're not worrying about how long you have been in a pose and also if you're concerned about falling asleep. If possible, I would suggest something that is not a severe sound. I like to use a timer from an app called Insight Timer as it has a number of sounds you can choose from – I use a bell chime. There are other similar apps out there too, so this may be something to consider if you have a smartphone. (This is one way your smartphone can be a force for good!)

Relaxed breath

Start by observing your breath, without trying to modify it. For instance, do you notice that your breath is shallow or choppy? Simply observing in this way can be helpful as a means of checking in with yourself. From here, guide your breath towards an even, relaxed breath where your inhale is about the same length as your exhale. Slowly count to four as you inhale, then slowly count to four as you exhale. This is known as 1:1 breathing or sama vritti in Sanskrit – 'sama' meaning 'balanced' or 'equal' and 'vritti' meaning 'fluctuation' or 'wave'. It is a calming breath. If you find that a count of four feels challenging for your breath capacity, then start with a lower count – inhale for two, exhale for two – and over time gradually move towards that slow count of four. Sama vritti is a wonderful practice that can be done on its own too. Later in this book you will find more breathing practices that can be done along with your restorative poses or on their own.

Worried about silence?

If silence feels too much, you might like to choose a piece of music or a sound that is soothing to you – for example, white noise – to play in the background. This could become a part of your practice ritual where you associate a particular sound or song(s) with your rest practice. We are all individuals so some of us will prefer to practise with music or sounds and some of us will prefer to practise in silence. My preference is to practise without music or background noise other than the sounds that are naturally in my environment. That said, if you do practise with music or sound, I would suggest, when you feel ready, you try practising with silence and see how that feels for you. You may find that moving away from music or sound to your breath being where your awareness goes makes for a deeper experience.

A practice journal

Related to this, if you're someone who likes to track things, you may wish to have a notebook nearby for immediately after your practice, where you can jot down any notes about your experience – for example, how a pose felt, whether you were warm enough, should you have worn socks and didn't. All of these things can be used to inform your practice in the future. You may also find that you have a light bulb moment about something in your life as you emerge from practice, in which case having a notepad and pen within easy reach to write that down before it has a chance to slip out of your head is something you will be grateful for.

Be kind to your mind

Yoga is a slowing down of the fluctuations of the mind
(Yoga Sutra 1.2, Patanjali)

Even after you've done everything you can to ensure your physical body is as comfortable as possible, mind chatter – the fluctuations of the mind referred to above – is real. Our brains are designed to think, so it's normal for the mind to wander. The practice of yoga can remind us that we are not our thoughts and can lead us to mental peace by witnessing, but not reacting or becoming attached to, thoughts.

When you come into a restorative yoga posture, don't be surprised if you find your mind is still very active while your body is still. Stillness can open up the space for the things we have been avoiding or worrying about to race to the forefront of our thoughts. We tend to think of this as a bad thing – often our response to discomfort is to distract ourselves. However, we can't resolve what we don't acknowledge. In restorative yoga postures we allow ourselves to be still. When we are still, this provides the space and opportunity to sit with discomfort until we are able to process it.

Rather than trying to push thoughts away, resolve to be kind to yourself. If you're using sound, gently guide your awareness to that each time thoughts arise. If practising in silence, then allow your relaxed breath to be your point of focus, so guide your awareness back to the rise and fall of your inhale and exhale each time a thought arises, or you can try a simple visualisation such as one of the following.

Cloud watching: Imagine you are lying on the grass. It's one of those gorgeous days when it feels as though the colour dial has been turned up on the world. All is vibrant. Maybe you even sense the smell of the grass or the soil. From your place on the grass, you are looking up at the beautiful clear blue sky. Each time a thought arises, it appears as brilliant white cloud that floats into your field of vision, and in the same way you observe that cloud float in, you watch the cloud float away, across the sky and out of your view. Each time a thought arises in the form of a cloud, you can simply observe that cloud for what it is and, without attachment, watch each cloud float away, out of your field of vision, allowing you to continue to enjoy your clear blue sky.

Thought trains: Imagine you're sitting on a bench on a train station platform. Each time a thought arrives in the form of a train, you can watch it pull into the station. You can observe what the train looks like, what colour it is, how many carriages it has. You might even observe other people getting on and off the train, but you don't need to get on because it's not your train. Then you can watch the train leave as it pulls away from the platform and goes on its way, knowing that you are OK and safe, sitting on the bench on the platform.

Move your energy

Sometimes, going straight from your daily activities into a restorative practice might feel like a challenge. In order to be able to settle into stillness, incorporating some gentle movements beforehand can be helpful. Ease yourself in by trying one or all of the following movements before you start your restorative yoga practice. Allow these movements to flow smoothly along with your breathing, so that you're moving mindfully without rushing. Only do as much as feels right for you, so that you're not forcing or straining, you're practising with kindness to yourself – practising with ahimsa.

Cat cow flow

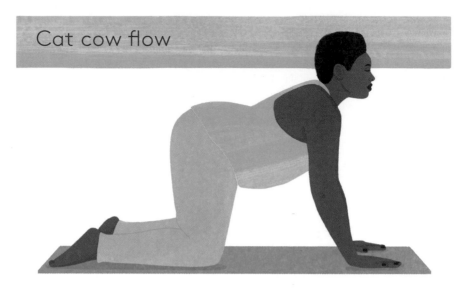

If practising on the floor, come to hands and knees in an all-fours position with your wrists in line with your shoulders and your knees in line with your hips. Start with your spine in its neutral position (this is when all three curves of the spine – neck (cervical), upper/middle (thoracic) and lower (lumbar) – are in their natural position). Inhale. As you exhale, round your upper back (like a cat rounding its back – Cat pose). As you inhale, guide your spine back to neutral and then arch your spine into a gentle backbend, so that your tailbone lifts slightly up to the ceiling, your belly drops downward and your

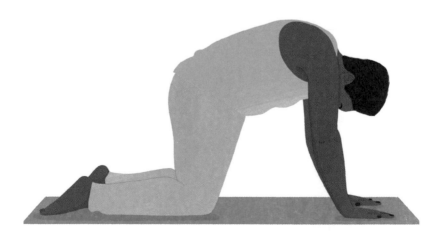

gaze lifts slightly. Let your shoulder blades slide down, away from your ears (cow pose). Repeat this for five to 10 breaths, linking your movement to your breathing rhythm. If you have discomfort in your knees, place a folded blanket or similar under your knees for padding. If you have discomfort in your wrists, either make fists with your hands and rest on your knuckles rather than palms, or come on to your forearms.

If practising on a chair, sit at the front of your chair seat to allow your spine to come into a neutral position (this is because sitting back in your chair is likely to cause you to slouch and makes sitting up more challenging). Ensure that the soles of your feet are flat on the floor or another flat surface and rest your hands palms-down on your thighs. Inhale. As you exhale, roll back on your pelvis. This will allow the upper back to round. Let your shoulders round forward and your chin move in towards your chest. As you inhale, guide your spine back to neutral and roll forward on your pelvis. This will create a gentle backbend, with your belly moving forward. Let your shoulders move back and down and your chest and gaze lift slightly. Repeat this for five to 10 breaths, linking your movement to your breathing rhythm.

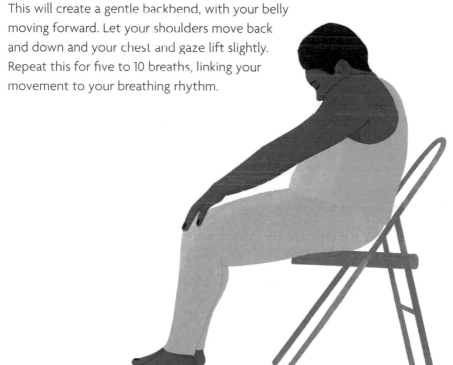

Seated torso circles

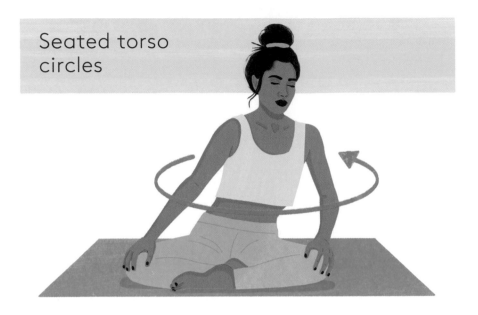

If practising on the floor, sit in a cross-legged position. Rest your hands palms-down on your knees. As you inhale, move your upper body forward. As you exhale, circle your upper body to your right, behind you, and then to your left until you come back to centre where you started. As you draw these circles with your body, allow your pelvis and spine to move as they need to, so that your movement is fluid. As your upper body moves back, allow your spine to round and the chin to tuck in slightly. As your upper body moves forward, allow the centre of your chest to lead the movement. Continue with these circles to the right for five to 10 breaths, allowing your circles to be as small or large as feels good for your body. Repeat, circling your torso to the left.

    If practising on a chair, sit at the front of your chair seat to allow your spine to come into a neutral position. Ensure that the soles of your feet are flat on the floor or another flat surface and rest your hands palms-down on your thighs. As you inhale, move your upper body forward. As you exhale, circle your body to the right and all the way around in a circle until you reach back to the centre where you started (same as described for if doing this movement sitting on the floor). Take five to 10 circles around to the right. Repeat, circling your torso around to the left.

Windscreen wipers

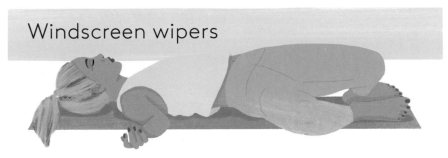

If practising lying on the floor, lie down on your back with your knees bent and the soles of your feet on the surface you're resting on. Toe-heel your feet apart until your feet and knees are wider than your hip distance and turn your feet out slightly, allowing your knees to be in line with your toes. Rest your arms out to your sides (at approximately shoulder height), either keeping them straight with your palms facing up, or with your elbows bent and palms facing up to form a 'cactus shape' with your arms.

Inhale. As you exhale, allow both knees to gently fall over to your right. As you inhale, bring your knees back to centre. On your next exhale, allow both knees to fall over to your left. Bring your knees back to centre as you inhale. Continue with this five to 10 times on each side, linking your breath to your movement. As your knees move to the right and left, they might touch the floor or surface you're lying down on, but they don't have to. Allow this movement to be as small or as big as feels right for you.

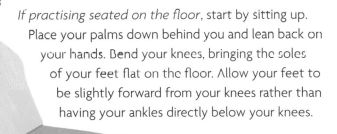

If practising seated on the floor, start by sitting up. Place your palms down behind you and lean back on your hands. Bend your knees, bringing the soles of your feet flat on the floor. Allow your feet to be slightly forward from your knees rather than having your ankles directly below your knees.

Toe-heel your feet apart so that your feet and knees are wider than your hip distance and let your toes turn out slightly.

Inhale. As you exhale, allow both knees to gently fall over to your right. As you inhale, bring your knees back to centre. On your next exhale, allow both knees to gently fall over to your left. As you inhale, bring your knees back to centre. Continue with this five to 10 times on each side, linking your breath to your movement. As with the supine version of this, as your knees move to the right and left, they might touch the floor, but they don't have to. Allow this movement to be as small or as big as feels right for you.

Seated twist

As an alternative to Windscreen wipers, you could try this Seated twist. Sit at the front of your chair seat to allow your spine to come into a neutral position. Ensure that the soles of your feet are flat on the floor. Rest your right hand on your left thigh and place your left hand on the side or back of the chair. As you inhale, keeping your chin parallel to the ground, lengthen the crown of your head upwards, sitting taller. As you exhale, gently rotate your upper body to your right. Either keep your chin in line with your breastbone or turn your head to look over your right shoulder. If you are turning your head do so gently – less is more. If turning your head causes your breathing to feel restricted, allow your chin to stay in line with your breastbone.

Stay in your twist to your right for two to three breaths. When you feel ready to release your twist, bring your body back to centre on an exhale. Repeat your twist to your left.

Seated side bend

If practising on a chair, sit towards the front of your chair seat to allow your spine to come into a neutral position. Ensure that the soles of your feet are flat on the floor or another flat surface.

Rest your left hand either on your left thigh or hold on to the left side of your chair. As you inhale, reach your right arm up towards the sky. As you exhale, reach your upper body over to your left, so that you're stretching the right side of your torso. Allow your right hip to stay down on the chair seat and your right shoulder to move down away from your right ear. Inhale to reach back up towards the sky, exhale as you place your right hand down on your right thigh or hold on to the right side of your chair. On your next inhale, reach your left arm up towards the sky and, as you exhale, reach your left arm and upper body over to your right, so that you're stretching the left side of your torso. Allow your left hip to stay down on the chair seat and your left shoulder to move down away from your left ear. Inhale to reach back up towards the sky, exhale as you place your left hand down on your left thigh or hold on to the left side of your chair. Repeat this five to 10 times on each side.

If practising on the floor, sit up with a neutral spine. Sitting up on a cushion or two can help you to achieve this, especially if you find your back rounding while you're seated. A tip if using cushions here is to sit on the corner rather than the flat side of the cushion(s) – this will help tilt your pelvis forward, allowing your spine to be in its neutral position.

Place your left hand down on the floor beside you. As you inhale, reach your right arm out to your right and up towards the sky, and, as you exhale, reach your right arm and upper body over to your left, so that you're stretching the right side of your torso. Allow your right hip to stay grounded and your right shoulder to move down away from your right ear. Inhale to reach back up towards the sky, exhale as you place your right hand down on the floor beside you. On your next inhale, reach your left arm out to your left and up towards the sky, and, as you exhale, reach your left arm and upper body over to your right, so that you are stretching the left side of your torso. Allow your left hip to stay grounded and your left shoulder to move down away from your left ear. Inhale to reach back up towards the sky, exhale as you place your left hand down by your side. Repeat this five to 10 times on each side.

Tense and release

If you usually experience muscle spasms or have a specific back condition, then check with your doctor whether the following is suitable for you, but another way to help the body get ready to relax is to tense the muscles and then release them.

One way you can do this is to start by bringing your awareness to your breathing. Inhale and exhale a few times, allowing your breath to be steady. On your next inhale, clench your fists, toes, jaw and tense every muscle in your body that you can – squeeze and hold for one ... two ... three ... and then exhale to release everything. Repeat this three more times. Then allow your body to be heavy and return to a comfortable breathing rhythm.

Another approach is to, again, begin by bringing your awareness to your breathing. Inhale and exhale a few times. On your next inhale, make a fist with your right hand and tense your whole right arm – squeeze and hold. Then on an exhale, release your right arm and hand. On an inhale, make a fist with your left hand and tense your whole left arm – squeeze and hold. Then on an exhale, release your left arm and hand. On an inhale, scrunch your right toes and tense your whole right leg, including your right gluteal muscles – squeeze and hold. On an exhale, release your right foot and leg. On an inhale, scrunch your left toes and tense your whole left leg, including your left gluteal muscles. On an exhale, release your left foot and leg. On an inhale, tense your abdomen – squeeze and hold. On an exhale, release all tension in your abdomen. On an inhale, tense your chest – squeeze and hold. On an exhale, release all tension in your chest. On an inhale, tense your shoulders, taking them all the way up to your ears — squeeze and hold. On an exhale, completely release your shoulders. On an inhale, tense your whole face, head and neck, including your jaw — squeeze and hold. On an exhale, release all tension in your face, head, neck and jaw. Allow your whole body to be heavy and return to a comfortable breathing rhythm.

Savasana – the foundation of restorative yoga

This is the foundation, the root of all the other restorative poses. If there is only one pose you can do, then this is the one. As I mentioned earlier, this is what I did for 20 minutes a day every day for a whole year. If the most you can manage on any given day is two to three minutes, that's OK! You will still benefit from pausing and resting for this time. (Remember, 'Some is better than none'.) If you can manage 20 minutes, here is why it can be so beneficial for deep relaxation and rejuvenation:

- physiological relaxation, which is when we move from a sympathetic nervous system (SNS) state to a parasympathetic nervous system (PNS). The weight of the physical body completely lets go into the props or surface supporting it. Although we're all different, for the average person it can take around 15 minutes to make that shift.
- pratyahara, which translates as 'withdrawal of the senses', the fifth of Patanjali's eight limbs of yoga (see p. 19). This is a state where you're not disturbed. It is a stage between being awake and asleep. You may be aware of sounds around you, but you're not disturbed by them.

A deeply restorative savasana tends to be around 20 minutes to allow plenty of time to switch to a PNS state and have at least five minutes in this pratyahara state. This is a state that we may not get to experience unless engaging in a practice such as yoga nidra (more on this later in this book).

What I have discovered when I practise savasana for 20 minutes, and have also heard from the countless testimonials of students, is that in the beginning your mind will wander or race (thinking about dinner or your to-do list is common). At first the physical body is a little fidgety, but then at some point it's as though the weight of the body sinks down and the thinking mind goes somewhere else. However, it's not until the timer goes off at the end of practice that it's apparent the mind has been elsewhere and, at the same time, the physical body feels rejuvenated and muscle tension is eased. It's akin to being asleep, but not the same; it's a state that is incredibly difficult to describe and can only be experienced.

The five layers

For a little more understanding on the pratyahara state and what you might experience, not only in a restorative savasana, but also during a restorative pose or sequence when you're engaging in a practice of 20 minutes or more, it can be helpful to have an awareness that from a yoga perspective we are more than our physical body. Here's a short overview of the koshas – the five layers or 'sheaths' that you may move through or between during a practice.

The practice of restorative yoga is simple, yet it can be incredibly profound. Even to this day, it continues to teach me. All of the occasions when I think I have no time to practise, by lying down on the floor with my props I find that afterwards I am more clear-headed and efficient at completing those things that need to be done. In other words, making the time to practise savasana or any restorative pose (even if it's not for as long as 20 minutes) gives rather than takes time.

THE KOSHAS

The physical body (annamaya kosha) is what you will initially be aware of in restorative yoga poses, particularly the parts of the body in contact with the surfaces they're resting on, such as the floor, the bed, pillows, blankets, cushions and so on.

The energy body (pranamaya kosha) is enhanced by breathing practices – 'prana' translates as 'life force' and breath is one of the vehicles for transporting prana through the body (see the *CALM* section for more on this).

The mind/emotion body (manomaya kosha) incorporates the whole nervous system, including the brain. Sensory withdrawal (the 'pratyahara' state mentioned earlier) is rejuvenating for this layer. This place of sensory withdrawal can also be reached via yoga nidra or 'yogic sleep' (see the *CALM* section for more on this). Deep rest and deep sleep regenerates the mind/emotion body.

The wisdom body (vijnanamaya kosha) represents our discernment. Stillness – restorative yoga in this instance, but also yoga nidra and sitting meditation – strengthens our ability to connect to our inner wisdom and have clarity of judgement. Think of times in your life when you have made decisions in a tired, overwhelmed or highly stressed state. Would you have made a different decision if you had felt rested and had greater clarity of mind? By tending to the wisdom body, another by-product in day-to-day life can be the ability to pause before reacting when faced with difficult situations.

The bliss body (anandamaya kosha) is the fifth and final layer. 'Ananda' translates as 'bliss' or 'ecstasy'. It is our true nature, our essence. It is coming home to yourself. There is no a guarantee that you will experience moving through the layers during your practice to reach the bliss body. If you do, it is usually not until you end your practice that you have an awareness that you have 'been somewhere'. It is not something that you can force or 'will' to happen.

Supported restorative savasana

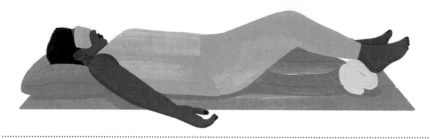

DURATION: 2 to 20 minutes
SUGGESTED PROPS: One cushion, one or two blankets, two bed pillows, one soft towel rolled into a long sausage shape, one soft scarf or eye mask

HOW TO GET THERE: If you're using music or a background sound, turn this on first (*see* pp. 21–2 for more on using sound).

Once you have decided where you will practise, before you lie down put a cushion in place to support your head and neck.

Carefully lie down on your back and slide your pillows underneath the backs of your knees, before extending your legs out straight over them. You can allow your legs to relax and your feet to roll outwards here. Having sufficient support under the knees is kinder on the lower back. This is particularly important to bear in mind if you experience back pain or have concerns around your lower back.

If you find that your heels don't touch the floor, take a rolled-up soft towel (or similar) and place it under your ankles for support.

Ensure your head and neck feel comfortable. If you notice that your chin is pointing upward (which can be triggering for your nervous system), then bring your chin inward towards your chest so that the back of your neck is lengthened. (What is happening in the cervical spine – the neck – can impact what is happening in the lumbar spine – the lower back – so the positioning of your head and neck is worth paying particular attention to, especially if you know that you have concerns around your lower back.)

Set your timer for your allotted time (for example, if you're allowing

20 minutes, then it's a good idea to set your timer now for 22 minutes so that you have time to settle into your pose).

Cover your body with a blanket or throw.

If you're using an eye cover, cover your eyes.

Rest your arms by your sides with your palms facing up. Allow your hands to relax. You will notice that your fingers will naturally curl in towards your palms. If placing your arms by your sides doesn't feel comfortable, try resting your palms down on your lower abdomen.

Before you completely settle into your supported restorative savasana, allow 20 to 30 seconds to see how you feel. Is there anything you can do to make yourself even 10 per cent more comfortable? Make any adjustments you need to until you no longer have the desire to move.

Guide your awareness to your breathing. First notice how your breath is doing, then gradually smooth out your breathing until your inhale is approximately the same length as your exhale (1:1 breathing/sama vritti).

Allow yourself to be here in your supported restorative savasana until your timer lets you know your practice has come to an end.

If you don't feel comfortable lying on flat on your back, the following are three alternatives.

Side-lying relaxation pose

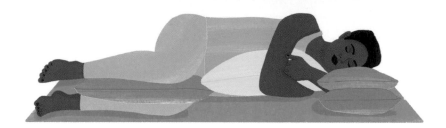

Side-lying relaxation pose can be practised during pregnancy, when lying on the back is no longer comfortable or advisable (usually after 20 weeks), but for circulatory reasons for parent and baby, it's important to lie on the left side of the body. Side-lying relaxation pose can also be practised shortly after eating and lying on the left side may ease digestion. In addition, this can be a good sleeping position to try if you find sleeping on your back in bed uncomfortable, particularly if you have been experiencing back pain. According to Ayurveda ('the science of life', which is often referred to as yoga's sister science), sleeping on the left side of the body can support the efficiency of the lymphatic system and research suggests that sleeping on the side of the body as opposed to the back or front may help the body process waste chemicals from the brain more effectively.

DURATION: 2 to 20 minutes
SUGGESTED PROPS: One or two cushions, one or two bed pillows, one or two blankets, one soft scarf or eye mask

HOW TO GET THERE: If you're using music or background sound, turn this on first. Then set your timer.

Lying down on your left side, place one or two cushions under the left side of your head. Ensure your cushions rest all the way into the curve where your neck meets your left shoulder.

Bend your knees to a 45- to 90-degree angle and place a pillow between your knees – this can help to keep your hips in line and avoid any uncomfortable pulling sensations around the lower back area.

Extend your left arm straight in front of you on the surface you are resting on, with left palm facing up. Make any adjustments to ensure your left shoulder feels settled – this might mean reaching your left arm a little further forward. If you feel as though your left arm would benefit from some support, place a folded blanket underneath your left arm.

If covering your eyes, you can drape your soft scarf over the side of your head so that it falls over your eyes. Or, if using a sleep mask, place it over your eyes.

From here you can either rest your right arm on your right side, with your right palm resting lightly on your tummy, or wrap both arms around your second pillow, hugging this pillow close to your body.

If you would like to cover your body with a blanket or equivalent, please do so and then make any adjustments you need to before settling in to rest here until your timer lets you know that your practice has come to an end.

SIDE-LYING RELAXATION DURING PREGNANCY

During pregnancy, practising side-lying relaxation on the left and sleeping on the left is recommended as there is less likelihood of the foetus compressing the inferior vena cava. An important role of this large vein that runs along the right side of the spine is to return blood to the heart from the lower part of the body. Therefore, compression of the inferior vena cava can reduce the amount of blood returned to the heart, consequently impacting the levels of blood oxygen for both parent and baby (for more options during pregnancy, see pp. 97–101).

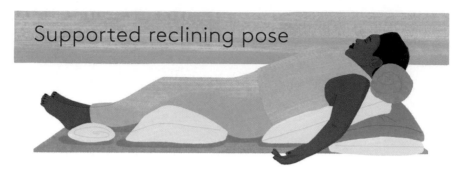

Supported reclining pose

In this pose, the upper body is propped up slightly. It may be helpful if you don't want to lie flat on your back or if you would like to avoid falling asleep.

DURATION: 2 to 20 minutes

SUGGESTED PROPS: Two or three pillows, one or two cushions, one or two blankets, one soft towel rolled into a sausage shape, one soft scarf or eye mask

HOW TO GET THERE: If you're using music or background sound, turn this on first. Then set your timer.

Create an incline with one or two pillows and a cushion by placing a cushion underneath one of the short ends of your pillow(s). The higher end is where your head will rest when you lie down.

Sit with your tailbone at the lower end of the pillow/cushion set-up.

Place a pillow under the backs of your knees. Under your ankles place your soft rolled-up towel.

Lie back on to your pillow/cushion set-up so that your upper body is supported. Ensure that your head and neck feel comfortable. If your chin is pointing upwards here, it is advisable to place some extra support under the head to allow the chin to be positioned slightly inwards towards the chest).

If you are covering your body, use a blanket or equivalent to cover up.

If you are covering your eyes, place your scarf or mask over your eyes.

See where feels comfortable to rest your arms – for example, by your sides with your palms facing up or palms-down on your lower abdomen.

Make any adjustments you need to before settling in to rest here until your timer lets you know that your practice has come to an end.

Seated savasana

DURATION: 2 to 20 minutes
SUGGESTED PROPS: One chair, one or two bed pillows or one or two cushions, one or two blankets, one soft scarf or eye mask (optional: two hardback books to rest your feet on)

HOW TO GET THERE: Please ensure your chair is on a non-slip surface and positioned in such a way that it will not move while you're in your savasana.

Have all the props you would like to use within easy reach (depending on the chair you're sitting on, you might wish to sit on a cushion or a folded blanket for extra comfort).

Sitting upright in your chair, ensure that the soles of your feet are well supported (either on the floor or another stable surface) and that your back feels supported – this is where you might wish to add a pillow(s) or cushion(s) behind your back.

If you would like to cover up your body (partially or completely) with a blanket and to cover your eyes, do so here.

Rest your hands with your palms upwards on your thighs with your fingers gently curling inwards. Alternatively, rest a cushion or pillow on your abdomen and/or thighs and rest the backs of your hands on top.

Make any adjustments you need to before settling in to rest until your timer lets you know that your practice has come to an end.

When you're ready to exit this pose, pause for several breaths and allow yourself as much time as you need before gently moving on.

Seven days of savasana

This is the homework I set for yoga teacher trainees on the course I lectured on for eight years. There were always incredible insights as a result. I feel this is such a valuable exercise that I'm sharing it with you here, so that you can try it for yourself.

1   Try each of the savasana variations detailed above and pick your favourite. This will be the pose you practise.
2   Decide if there is a particular time of day you would like to practise and, if possible, stick with that time over the course of the seven days. However, don't worry if you need to practise at a different time each day.
3   Gather your props together, including your timer.
4   Have a notebook and pen nearby so that, if you want to, you can write down any observations or insights after each practice.
5   For seven consecutive days practise the savasana variation of your choice for 20 minutes. If 20 minutes feels too long, start with a time duration that you feel you can do and work your way up to as close to 20 minutes as possible. Even if you think you can't do 20 minutes, set your timer for this duration and give yourself permission to end your practice sooner if you wish. You may be surprised to find that once you're comfortable and settled, your body and mind will happily rest for longer than you initially expected.

The restorative yoga poses

Here are some of the restorative yoga poses that I teach most often and have found most effective for my students. I've included the fundamentals, plus some extras and variations that you can mix and match. I hope you'll find some favourites here that you'll return to again and again. Each of these poses can be practised alone or as part of a sequence. You'll find a range of sequences later, but here is a little more detail about the main poses you'll find in this book.

If you're using music or background sound, turn this on first. Likewise, if you are using a timer, set this before you settle into the pose.

A note about suggested props

For each of the poses detailed below, there are suggested props listed. You may not need every item mentioned for the pose described, but these suggestions are to help you envision how what you have available in your surroundings could be used and encourage you to experiment with different items for performing the same function. For instance, two rolled-up or folded blankets – one supporting each hip in a pose – might feel more comfortable to you than using two cushions or two bed pillows to do the same thing. Or it may be that you feel better using a folded blanket to support your head in a reclining position rather than a cushion.

In the case of using a belt for support, this could be the belt from a dressing gown tied to form a loop or a belt with a buckle might be from a pair of jeans or a dress. A resistance band tied in a loop can work in a similar way, but will stretch a little more. Experimenting with your props in this way helps to make the practice your own, as well as helping to cultivate more awareness of what feels good for you. Some days you might feel that your body wants more or less support in certain places, so the prop suggestions here are not prescriptive. What's important is that you do use support where you need it.

Supported bound angle pose

DURATION: 1 to 5 minutes
SUGGESTED PROPS: Three to four cushions or bed pillows and/or two blanket rolls or towel rolls, an extra blanket to cover up with (optional: access to a wall)

HOW TO GET THERE: If you feel that you would benefit from extra support for your back, you may wish to sit against a wall.

Place a cushion(s) (or pillows or folded blankets) on the floor to sit on. This will elevate your hips to allow your spine to be in a neutral position (not rounding forward through the back), as well as providing support for your sitting bones and alleviating lower back discomfort. Sitting on a corner rather than a flat side of your cushion(s) or blanket(s) may help you achieve this more easily.

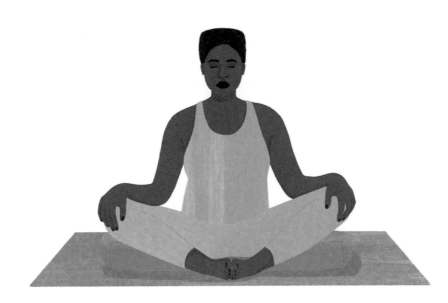

Bring the soles of your feet together, so that your knees fall to either side, forming a diamond shape with your legs. To ensure that there is no strain on the hips or knees, place cushions (or equivalent such as blanket rolls, towel rolls or bed pillows) under each leg. If you have been experiencing any knee discomfort, try adding more support here and moving the feet further forward so that there is a larger space between your heels and pelvis.

Either close your eyes or soften your gaze to one spot to allow the muscles around your eyes to be as relaxed as possible. If you would like to block out the light, then you have the option to cover your eyes with a soft scarf and tie it lightly at the back of your head to keep it in place. You could also use a sleep mask here if you have one. If your jaw feels tight, parting your lips slightly can help.

Allow your arms and hands to rest where they feel most comfortable for you   this might be with your palms down or up on your legs or gently resting your hands in your lap.

Make any final adjustments you need to before settling in, noting whether you would like to add any extra support or not, so that you are able to be here for your chosen duration with as much ease and comfort as possible.

When you feel ready to exit your supported bound angle pose, bring your hands to the outside of each thigh, using your hands to move your knees towards each other until the soles of your feet are flat on the surface where you have been resting. Extend both legs out straight in front of you. Feel free to add some gentle movement such as circling your ankles one way and then the other.

Chair-supported bound angle pose – version A

DURATION: 2 to 5 minutes
SUGGESTED PROPS: Two chairs, two or three bed pillows, two or three cushions, one or two blankets, one soft scarf or eye mask (optional: one belt or resistance band, two hardback books)

HOW TO GET THERE: For this and any other pose involving chairs, please ensure your chairs are on a non-slip surface and positioned in such a way that they will not move during your practice. Likewise, it is not advisable to use chairs on wheels.

Have all the props you would like to use within easy reach. Sit in one chair with the opposite chair facing you. Depending on the chair you are sitting on, you might wish to sit on a cushion or a folded blanket for extra comfort.

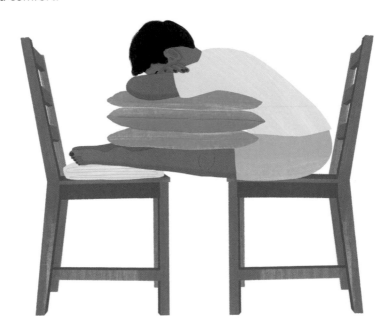

Place your feet on the chair seat in front of you. Bring the soles of your feet together and allow your knees to fall to either side, creating a diamond shape with your legs. If you feel your feet and ankles would benefit from padding, then keep a cushion or folded blanket on the chair seat.

If your hips feel particularly tight and/or would benefit from extra support, this is where a dressing gown belt (or similar) or something stretchy like a resistance band may be useful:

* Tie the ends of your belt or resistance band together securely to form a loop. The size of the loop will depend on the proportions of your body.
* Create a figure-eight shape with your loop.
* With your legs in your bound angle shape, place each loop over each knee. This is where you will notice whether you would like to make your loop smaller or larger to provide the right amount of support for you. A smaller loop will provide greater support if your hips feel particularly tight.

If you would like to stay sitting upright in your bound angle pose:

* There is an option to cover up with a blanket and cover your eyes.
* Rest your palms on your lower abdomen and guide your awareness to the rise and fall of your breathing.
* There is an option to practise diaphragmatic breathing here (see Breathing practices in the CALM section).

If you would like to come into a forward bend in your Bound angle pose:

* Place your stacked pillows in front of you so that one end rests on your feet and the other end is close to your pelvis.
* Bring your upper body forward on to the pillows (stack your pillows up with a cushion – as with Supported child's pose – if you would like to add some extra height).
* If you would like to cover up, place a blanket over the back of your body. This could be folded so that it covers just your lower back and

hips, or it could be opened out to completely cover the back of your body.

- Place one forearm on top of the other and rest your forehead there. Allow your chin to tuck slightly in towards your chest.
- Guide your awareness to the rise and fall of your breathing.
- There is an option to practice 1:1 breathing (sama vritti) or 1:2 breathing here (*see Breathing practices* in the *CALM* section).

When you're ready to exit this pose, if you're using a belt or resistance band remove this first. Carefully move your feet off your second chair and then rest the soles of your feet flat on the floor (or an alternative surface such as two hardback books). Pause here for a few breaths before moving on.

Chair-supported bound angle pose – version B

This variation requires less propping and is also an option if your hips feel especially tight or your mobility does not allow you to rest your feet on a chair in front of you.

DURATION: 2 to 5 minutes
SUGGESTED PROPS: One chair, two or three bed pillows or two or three cushions (use more if needed), one or two blankets, one soft scarf or eye mask (optional: one belt or resistance band, two hardback books)

HOW TO GET THERE: Stack your pillows or cushions on top of each other on the floor in front of the chair you will be sitting in. If you would like to pad the seat of the chair you will be using, add a folded blanket or extra cushion here.

Sit towards the front of your chair seat to help your spine come into a neutral position. If this is not possible, add support to your back to help you sit up as straight as you can. Rest the outside edges of your feet on your pillows or cushions on the floor, bringing the soles of your feet together and allowing your knees to move out to either side into a bound angle shape.

If you would like extra support for your hips, follow the steps for using a belt or resistance band described in Chair-supported bound angle – version A.

Before settling in here you have the option to cover up by resting a blanket over your lap and/or wrapping a blanket over your shoulders.

If you would like to cover your eyes you can do so with a soft scarf tied lightly at the back of your head, or use a sleep mask.

When you're ready, you can exit this pose in the same way as Chair-supported bound angle – version A.

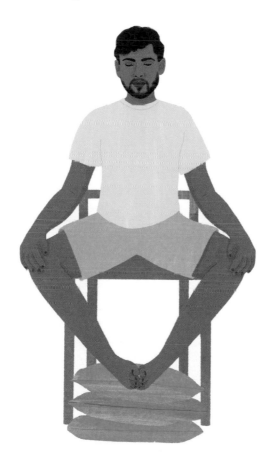

Supported reclining bound angle pose

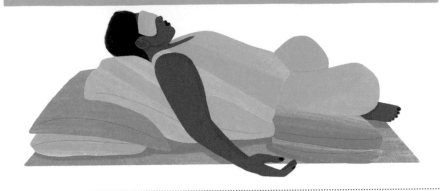

DURATION: 5 to 20 minutes
SUGGESTED PROPS: One to three pillows, one to three cushions, one or two blankets, one soft scarf or eye mask

HOW TO GET THERE: Create an incline with one or two bed pillows and a cushion by placing a cushion underneath one of the short ends of your pillow(s) so that one end is higher than the other. The higher end is where your head will rest when you lie down.

Sit with your tailbone at the lower end of the pillow/cushion set-up.

Place the soles of your feet together and allow your knees to fall out to either side so that your legs form a diamond shape.

Either slide a pillow underneath your legs so that the outside of each knee is supported or place a cushion, or blanket or towel rolls, under each knee. This will provide more ease for the knees and hips in this position.

Lie back on to your pillow/cushion set-up so that your upper body is supported. Ensure that your head and neck feel comfortable. If your chin is pointing upwards here, it is advisable to place some extra support, such as a cushion or folded blanket, under the head to allow the chin to be positioned slightly inwards towards the chest.

If you are covering your body, use a blanket or equivalent to cover up.

If you are covering your eyes, place your soft scarf, sleep mask or eye pillow over your eyes.

See where it feels comfortable to rest your arms – for example, by your sides with your palms facing up or placing your palms down on your lower abdomen. If you have access to extra props such as two more cushions or two blanket rolls, then one placed on either side of your pillow/cushion incline can act as a support for each arm.

Make any adjustments you need to before settling in to rest here until your timer lets you know that your practice has come to an end.

When you're ready to exit your Supported reclining bound angle, bring your hands to the outside of each thigh, then use your hands to carefully bring your knees towards each other until the soles of your feet are flat on the surface where you have been resting. Place your palms down by your sides (either side of your hips), then press down on your palms to help you come slowly up to sitting without needing to twist your back on your way up. Extend both legs out straight in front of you. Feel free to add some gentle movement such as circling your ankles one way and then the other.

Supported reclining twist – version A

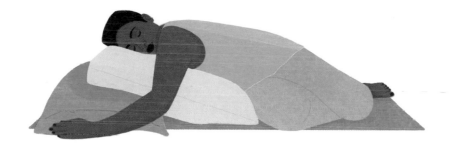

DURATION: 2 to 5 minutes
SUGGESTED PROPS: One to three pillows, one to three cushions, one or two blankets, one soft scarf or eye mask

HOW TO GET THERE: Create an incline with one or two bed pillows and a cushion by placing a cushion underneath one of the short ends of your pillow(s) so that one end is higher than the other. The higher end is where your head will rest when you lie down.

Sit with your tailbone at the lower end of the pillow/cushion set-up.

Keeping your knees bent, bring both knees over to your right side and allow your right hip to rest at the lower end of your pillow/cushion incline. Place a cushion, or an alternative such as a folded blanket(s), if you prefer, between your knees.

Turn your torso to your right, placing your hands on either side of your pillow/cushion incline.

As you inhale, lengthen the front of your body. As you exhale, ease your torso on to your pillow/cushion incline with your head at the higher end of your props. Ensure that your upper body feels fully supported. If you find that your head is dropping over the edge of your pillow(s), then slide your hips slightly back so that the side of your head can rest comfortably on your pillow(s).

If you're covering your body, use a blanket or equivalent to cover up.

If you would like to cover your eyes, drape your soft scarf over the side of your head so that it falls over your eyes or place your sleep mask over your eyes.

See where it feels comfortable to rest your arms – you could allow your arms to rest along either side of your pillow(s) or you could reach your arms around to the top of your pillow/cushion incline until you're hugging your pillow(s)/cushion. If you have access to extra props, such as two more cushions or two blanket rolls, then one placed on either side of your pillow/cushion incline can act as a support for each arm.

Stay here in your supported reclining twist for up to five minutes. When you're ready to change sides, carefully slide your hands back towards you along either side of your pillow(s) and press your palms down so that you can carefully lift your torso up away from your props.

Bring both knees over to your left to repeat your supported twist on the other side for the same duration.

Supported reclining twist – version B

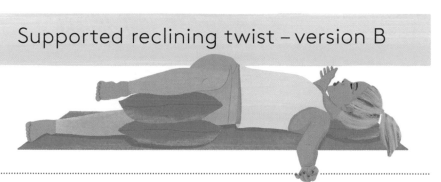

DURATION: 2 to 5 minutes
SUGGESTED PROPS: One to three cushions, one to three bed pillows, one blanket, one soft scarf or eye mask

HOW TO GET THERE: Lie down on your right-hand side with your legs stacked on top of each other. Place one or two bed pillows in front of your thighs lengthways (from hip to knee). Bend your left leg to approximately 90 degrees and rest your left leg on the pillows. If you feel any discomfort in your lower back, add another pillow under your left leg.

Place a cushion or pillow under the right side of your head for support. Ensure that the space from the top of the right side of your neck to your right shoulder is supported too.

Reach both arms in front of you at about shoulder height, with your left palm on top of your right palm. As you exhale, reach your left arm back towards the floor behind you so that your arms form one straight line with both palms facing up. You may wish to add a cushion or blanket roll under your left arm for support (this is certainly recommended if your left arm doesn't touch the ground or if you feel any discomfort in your left shoulder when reaching your left arm back).

See which way you would like to turn your head. Allowing your face to be in the same direction as your right arm or towards the ceiling is gentler, while turning your face towards your left arm would be a deeper twist. For some of us, a deeper twist might cause the breath to feel slightly restricted, in which case, opting to turn your head towards your right would be advisable.

Allow your abdomen to be soft. You might notice your navel gently rising and falling.

When you're ready to move out of your twist, bring your left palm back on to your right palm, carefully slide your left leg off your pillows and roll on to your back. Rest here on your back for a few breaths. While you're here you may wish to hug your knees into your chest and gently rock from side to side a few times. This rocking movement can provide a little massage for the back.

When you feel ready, roll on to your left side to repeat your twist, moving your pillows over to your left side with you to support your right leg this time.

Supported child's pose – version A

DURATION: 2 to 5 minutes
SUGGESTED PROPS: Two to three blankets (or two towels and one blanket/throw), two to three cushions (optional: two to three pillows, an eye cover such as a soft scarf, sleep mask or eye pillow)

HOW TO GET THERE: Come to kneeling. Place a folded blanket under your knees for padding if needed. A rolled-up towel or blanket under the tops of your feet can be helpful if this area feels tender in this position. Alternatively, if you're already kneeling on a blanket, you could squish the sides of this blanket under the tops of your feet.

If you find that you would like some padding between the backs of your thighs and calves, you could place a pillow or cushions here.

If you would like to cover up, place a blanket or equivalent over the back of your body, including your feet. You can choose whether you would like to cover up to the base of your neck or to place your blanket completely over your head to cocoon your whole body.

Without support for your torso, place one forearm on top of the other and rest your forehead there. If you would like padding for your forehead, you could place a soft scarf or eye pillow on top of your hands before lowering your forehead. If bringing your forehead down to your forearms feels too low or uncomfortable, then this is where a chair might be useful (see version B).

With support for your torso, stack two to three bed pillows on top of each other and place them lengthways in front of you. Bring your knees apart so that you can move the pillows as close to you as possible. Fold your upper body on to the pillows, resting one ear down. If you would like to elevate your head higher, place a cushion under the end of the pillows furthest away from you. This will create an incline where your head can rest at the higher end. If you have a soft scarf you may wish to drape it over the side of your head to cover your eyes. See where feels comfortable to rest your arms. You could allow your arms to rest along either side of your pillow(s) or you could reach your arms around to the top of your pillow/cushion incline until you're hugging your pillow(s)/cushion. If you have access to extra props such as two more cushions or two blanket rolls, then one placed on either side of your pillow stack/incline can act as support for each arm.

For vagus nerve stimulation (*see* p. 16) in Supported child's pose, the addition of a folded blanket resting at your hip creases and across the tops of your thighs can be very helpful. Utilised in this way, the blanket provides gentle compression to the abdomen and it can also ease menstrual cramps. If you do not have access to a blanket, try making fists with your hands and placing them at each hip crease before folding your upper body forward into your Supported child's pose.

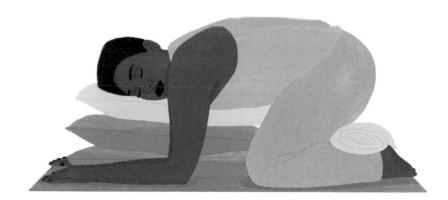

Supported child's pose – version B – chair variation

DURATION: 2 to 5 minutes

SUGGESTED PROPS: One chair, two to three blankets (or two towels and a blanket), two to three cushions (optional: two to three pillows, an eye mask)

HOW TO GET THERE: Follow all the steps to set up Supported child's pose – version A, and place a chair in front of you so that you're facing the chair seat. Position the chair close enough to your body so that you can rest your forehead on the chair seat, with your forearms on either side of your head. For extra height you could place one forearm on top of the other on the chair seat and rest your forehead on your arms. Feel free to use a blanket, cushion or pillow to add padding to the chair seat or your forearms.

If you have a third blanket or equivalent (such as a towel), you could fold it into a long rectangular shape and either place it over your hips and lower back to add some gentle weight to this part of the body, or place it at your hip crease and the tops of your thighs so that when you bring your upper body forward into your Supported child's pose the blanket gently compresses the lower abdomen.

When you're ready to exit this pose, carefully lift your head and upper body as you guide yourself up to a kneeling position. Pause here for a few breaths before moving on.

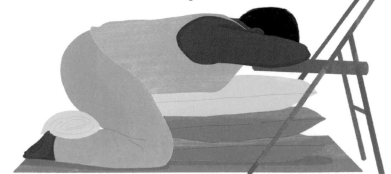

Supported child's pose – version C – two-chair variation

DURATION: 2 to 5 minutes

SUGGESTED PROPS: Two chairs, two or three bed pillows, two or three cushions, one or two blankets, one soft scarf or eye mask (optional: two hardback books if you need to elevate your feet)

HOW TO GET THERE: Have all the props you would like to use within easy reach. Sit in one chair with the other chair facing you. Depending on the chair you are sitting on, you might wish to sit on a cushion or a folded blanket for extra comfort.

If you're able to straddle the chair you're sitting on, this can create more ease when you come to bring your upper body forward. If you're not able to straddle the chair, allow your feet to be about hip distance apart to create some space. Ideally, the soles of both your feet will be flat on the ground.

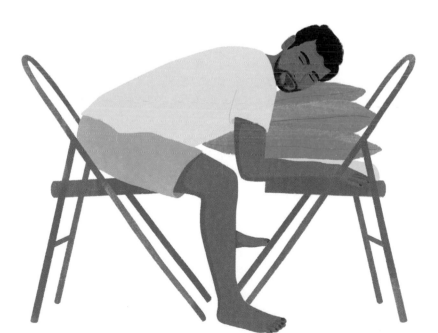

Otherwise, bring the floor up to your feet by placing them on a flat surface such as some hardback books. Place a cushion on the chair seat facing you and stack two to three pillows on top of each other lengthways on the cushion, creating an incline. Your head will be resting at the higher end.

Bring your upper body forward until your torso is resting on the pillows. If this feels like too much of a reach, then try stacking your pillows up higher with an extra cushion.

If you would like to cover up, place a blanket over the back of your body. This could be folded so that it covers just your lower back and hips, or it could be opened out to completely cover the back of your body.

Reach your arms around the sides of your pillows so that you're hugging them or rest your forearms down on the chair either side of the pillows. Rest one ear down on your pillows with your chin slightly tucking in towards your chest. If you would like to cover your eyes, drape your soft scarf over the side of your head so that it falls gently over your eyelids. Or if you're using a sleep mask instead, put it on.

When you feel ready, turn your head so that you're resting your opposite ear down on your pillows for a while too. Adjust your eye cover as necessary.

When you're ready to exit this pose, carefully hold on to the sides of your second chair and lift your upper body away from your pillows until you're sitting up tall. Pause here for a few breaths before moving on.

Try each of these versions of Supported child's pose and note what your experience is of each version to see if you have a favourite. You may even find that you would like to alternate between them each time you practise, depending on how you feel that day.

Face-down relaxation pose

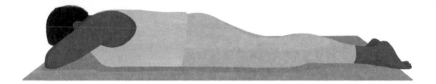

....

DURATION: 5 to 10 minutes
SUGGESTED PROPS: One or two pillows, one or two blankets, one soft scarf or eye mask

....

HOW TO GET THERE: Face-down relaxation pose can be practised prop-free or for extra comfort you can practise this with the addition of a blanket and optional elevation of the feet on pillows or a rolled-up blanket or towel.

For the prop-free version, lie face down on the surface where you are practising. Place one hand on top of the other and rest your forehead on the backs of your hands. Your feet can be hip distance or wider apart. Feel free to play with the positioning of your legs and feet until you're in a position where you feel so comfortable you have no desire to move.

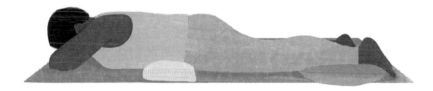

For the propped version, place one or two pillows (you may need two pillows stacked on top of each other if they're very thin) where your feet will be on the surface where you will be practising. Alternatively, you can roll up a blanket or equivalent into a long sausage shape.

Lie face down, placing your lower legs on your pillow(s) so that your feet gently drape over the edge and toes point down. If you're using a blanket roll instead here, place the tops of your feet over the blanket so that your ankles are supported and your toes point down.

If you would like to use a blanket or two to add some weight to your body, place a folded blanket(s) or equivalent over your hips and lower back.

For vagus nerve stimulation in Face-down relaxation pose, similar to the use of a folded blanket in Supported child's pose, the addition of a folded blanket on the abdomen can be very helpful for stimulating the vagus nerve. Fold a blanket into a long rectangular shape so that it fits between the base of your lower ribs and the tops of your hips. When you lie down on the blanket, to avoid lower back compression ensure that it doesn't press into your hip bones.

Place one hand on top of the other and rest your forehead on the backs of your hands. If you would like padding for your forehead, you could place a soft scarf or eye pillow on top of your hands before resting your forehead. An alternative way to use your scarf or eye pillow is to drape it on the back of your neck to add some gentle weight.

When you feel ready to transition out of this pose, slowly slide your hands alongside your shoulders, press your palms down on to the surface you're resting on and bring your hips back towards your heels. Pause here, then carefully guide yourself up to a comfortable kneeling or sitting position. Stay here for few breaths before moving on.

Supported half-frog pose

DURATION: 2 to 5 minutes on each side (up to 10 minutes in total)
SUGGESTED PROPS: One or two pillows, one or two blankets, one cushion, one soft scarf or eye mask

HOW TO GET THERE: Like Face-down relaxation pose, this can be practised with or without props.

For the prop-free version, lie face down on the surface where you're practising. Place one hand on top of the other and rest your forehead on the backs of your hands. You can either keep your forehead down or turn your head to one side. For either head position, allow your chin to tuck slightly in towards your chest to allow your neck to be in a more relaxed position.

Bend your right knee and slide your right leg along the floor to an approximately 90-degree angle. If you experience a pinching sensation in your right hip, bringing the sole of your right foot towards your left inside leg will change the angle of your right leg and should ease any discomfort.

When you feel ready to change legs, carefully extend your right leg back and slide your left leg out to your left side. Stay here for the same duration as you did with your right leg. If you were resting the side of your head on your hands, then turn your head to the other side now.

For the propped version, place one or two pillows (or two pillows stacked on top of each other if they're very thin) where your feet will be. Alternatively, you can roll up a blanket or towel into a long sausage shape.

Lie face down, placing your lower legs on your pillow(s) so that your feet gently drape over the edge and your toes point down. If you're using a blanket roll instead here, place the tops of your feet over the blanket so that your ankles are supported and your toes point down.

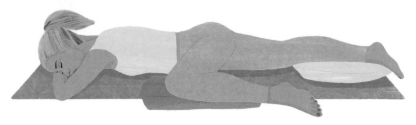

Place one hand on top of the other and rest your forehead on the backs of your hands. If you would like padding for your forehead, you could place a soft scarf or eye pillow on top of your hands before resting your forehead. Alternatively, drape it on the back of your neck to add some gentle weight.

Bend your right knee and slide your right leg along the floor to an approximately 90-degree angle. If you would like to pad your right knee and/ or ankle, place a pillow or cushion under your right leg. If you experience a pinching sensation in your right hip, bring the sole of your right foot towards your left inside leg, adjusting the position of your pillow/cushion accordingly.

For vagus nerve stimulation fold a blanket into a long rectangular shape so that it fits between the base of your lower ribs and the tops of your hips. Ensure that it doesn't press into your hip bones, to avoid lower back compression. If your blanket fold is long enough, then you can wrap the ends over your lower back if you like (this is a tip I learnt from Bo Forbes). Wrapping the blanket around the body can feel supportive and creates the comforting sensation of feeling held. Do give this a try to see if you like it.

When you feel ready to change legs, carefully extend your right leg back and slide your left leg out to your left side, bringing your pillow/cushion with you to pad your left leg if required. Stay here for the same duration as you did with your right leg. If you were resting the side of your head on your hands, then turn your head to the other side now.

When you feel ready to transition out of this pose (whichever version you are practising), carefully extend your left leg back so that both legs are behind you. If you were resting the side of your head on your hands, turn your head so that your forehead is resting down. Pause here in Face-down relaxation pose for a few breaths. When you feel ready to move again, slowly slide your hands alongside your shoulders, press your palms down on to the surface you are resting on and bring your hips back towards your heels. Pause here, then carefully guide yourself up to a comfortable kneeling or sitting position. Stay here for few breaths before moving on.

Supported fish pose – version A

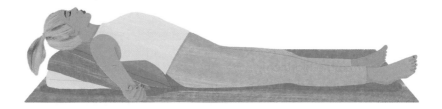

DURATION: 2 to 10 minutes
SUGGESTED PROPS: One to three pillows, one to three cushions,
one or two blankets, one soft scarf or eye mask

HOW TO GET THERE: Place your pillow(s) lengthways on to the surface
where you will be lying down. Create an incline with one or two bed pillows
and a cushion by placing a cushion underneath one of the short ends of
your pillow(s), so that one end is higher than the other. The higher end is
where your head will rest when you lie down.

Sit with your tailbone at the lower end of the pillow/cushion set-up.

Lie back on to your pillow/cushion set-up so that your upper body
is supported. Ensure your head and neck have enough support to feel as
comfortable as possible.

If you're covering your body, use a blanket or equivalent to cover up.

If you would like to cover your eyes, place a soft scarf, sleep mask or
eye pillow over your eyes.

When you're ready to transition from this pose, bend your knees and
bring the soles of your feet on to the surface you're resting on. Place your
palms by your hips and press your palms firmly down to help you come
up to sitting without needing to twist on your way up.

Supported fish pose – version B

DURATION: 2 to 5 minutes

SUGGESTED PROPS: Two or three pillows (or two or three blankets folded into a long rectangular shape), one or two cushions (or a folded blanket/blanket roll to support your head and neck), one soft scarf or eye mask

HOW TO GET THERE: Place a pillow horizontally on the surface you will be lying on (or up to three pillows stacked on top of each other if your pillows are thin, for added height). Your mid-upper back will be resting on your pillow(s).

Behind your pillow(s), place a cushion to support your head. Leave enough space between your pillow(s) and cushion for your shoulders.

Sit with your pillows behind you, soles of your feet on the surface you are resting on, and carefully lower yourself back until your mid and upper back are supported on your pillow(s) and your head is supported by your cushion.

Here, you have the option to rest the soles of your feet on the floor or extend your legs out straight. Keeping the soles of the feet flat on the floor will create a more stable position for the lower back. Extending the legs straight out will create more of a back bend and more of a stretch across the front of your body.

If you would like to cover up, place a blanket over your body.

If you would like to cover your eyes, place a soft scarf, sleep mask or eye pillow over your eyes.

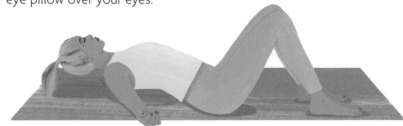

Use blankets instead – two to three folded into a long rectangular shape – if lying back over pillows feels too strong. If you are using blankets, which will be a lower height than pillows, you might find that you do not need a cushion for head support. Try with and without a cushion under your head to see what feels most comfortable for you.

When you feel ready to transition from your Supported fish pose, place the soles of your feet flat on to the surface you're resting on (if you're not there already). Carefully roll over, completely off your pillow(s) and cushion, on to one side. Rest on your side for a few breaths. When you're ready, guide yourself up to a comfortable sitting position. Pause here for several breaths before moving on.

Supported bridge pose

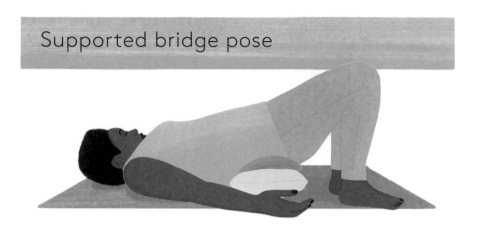

DURATION: 2 to 5 minutes

SUGGESTED PROPS: One or two pillows, one cushion, one or two blankets or four blankets (three folded, one to cover up), one soft scarf or eye mask (optional: one belt or a resistance band)

HOW TO GET THERE: Place your pillow(s) or folded blankets horizontally on to the surface where you will be lying down. If you're using more than one pillow, stack them on top of each other for added height. If using blankets, fold your blanket(s) into a long rectangular shape. If you're using more than one blanket, fold them all the same size so that they can neatly stack on top of each other.

Sit down on your pillow(s)/cushion. Adjust the positioning of your legs and feet so that they are approximately hip distance apart with your ankles in line with your knees and your feet parallel, toes facing forward. For extra support for your legs, you can tie a belt or resistance band around your legs at either mid-calf or mid-thigh level, whichever feels most comfortable for you. The use of a belt or similar here will help your legs remain hip distance apart with minimal effort and facilitate even more ease and relaxation in this pose. Ensure that the knot or buckle doesn't dig into your skin.

Place your palms down flat behind you so that your arms can support you as you lift your hips and slide them slightly forward of your pillow(s)/blanket(s). Lower your sacrum (the back of your pelvis, below your lower back curve) on to your pillow(s)/blanket(s). With the help of your arms, lower your upper body down until you are lying on your back, hips elevated on your pillow(s)/blanket(s), with knees bent and the soles of your feet flat on the surface you are resting on. Check that your legs and feet are still approximately hip distance apart with your feet parallel.

Notice how your head feels while you're lying down in your Supported bridge pose. If you feel you would benefit from more support here, place a cushion under your head. Allow your chin to be slightly tilted in towards your chest rather than towards the ceiling.

You have the option to add some gentle weight to the body here by resting a folded blanket across your abdomen, or open your blanket to cover up your body.

If you would like to cover your eyes, place a soft scarf or sleep mask over them.

Allow your arms and hands to rest where they feel most comfortable. Make any adjustments to ensure your shoulder blades feel settled on the surface you're resting on. Resting your arms back in a cactus shape (elbows bent, in line with your shoulders, and the backs of your arms and hands on the surface you're resting on) will create more of an open feeling across the upper chest and shoulders. Keeping your arms close by your sides will be gentler.

When you're ready to transition from this pose, press down through the soles of your feet until your hips lift off your pillow(s)/blanket(s). Carefully slide them behind your knees and lower your spine down so that your back is fully supported by the surface you're resting on. Let the backs of your knees rest on your pillow(s)/blanket(s). Visualise how the surface you're resting on is holding your body. Allow your whole body to be supported. You don't need to hold yourself up in any way. Rest here for several breaths before carefully bringing the soles of your feet on to your pillow(s)/blanket(s) and roll over to rest on one side. Carefully guide yourself up to a comfortable sitting position when you feel ready.

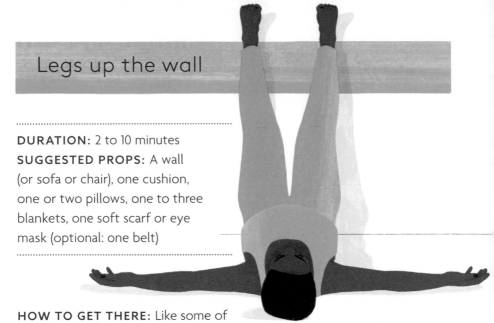

Legs up the wall

DURATION: 2 to 10 minutes
SUGGESTED PROPS: A wall
(or sofa or chair), one cushion,
one or two pillows, one to three
blankets, one soft scarf or eye
mask (optional: one belt)

HOW TO GET THERE: Like some of
the other poses, this can be practised with or without props.

For the prop-free version, you can practise using just the wall as follows.

Sit down on the floor (or bed, if practising there) with one hip alongside
the wall.

Carefully swing your legs and feet up on to the wall.

If your hamstrings feel particularly tight, try getting into Legs up the wall
by kneeling as close to the wall as possible with your back facing it. Lean
your upper body forward, carefully roll on to your back and swing your legs
and feet up on to the wall.

For whichever approach you choose, once you have your feet (heels)
touching the wall, you can choose how close the backs of your legs are
to the wall. Usually having your hips away from the wall (roughly 35 to
45 degrees) is gentler and less of a stretch along the back of the body
(especially the hamstrings, hips and lower back). Also, this position (with your
hips away from the wall) is preferable in terms of allowing your abdomen
and diaphragm to soften and therefore facilitating your breathing. Having
the backs of your legs and hips touching the wall (so that your body forms
more of a capital L shape) will usually create more of a stretching sensation
along the back of the body. With this in mind, please do adjust your hips to
a position in which you will be comfortable for a while by either shuffling

your hips closer to or further away from the wall.

When you feel ready to transition out of this pose, carefully bring the soles of your feet flat on to the wall and slide them down. Pause here for a few breaths before carefully rolling over to one side to rest there. When you feel ready, carefully guide yourself up to a comfortable sitting position.

For the propped version, for extra comfort and ease, place a blanket or equivalent on the surface your back and sacrum (back of the pelvis) will be resting on. You may wish to elevate your hips slightly by placing a pillow close to the wall. You could stack two pillows on top of each other here if your pillows are thin. Have a cushion or another pillow within your reach for head support.

Sit on your pillow(s) and carefully swing your legs and feet up the wall. Make any adjustments to the position of your hips and pillow(s) as needed. Place a cushion or pillow under your head for support if needed.

If you're using something like a dressing gown belt, which doesn't have a buckle, tie a knot in it to form a loop that is approximately your hip-width. Slide your feet through the loop and slide the belt up to either mid-calf height or mid thigh height (whichever feels most comfortable). If using a belt with a buckle, use the buckle to create a loop that is approximately your hip-width and follow the above steps. The benefit of using a belt is that it creates support for your legs by comfortably, yet securely, holding them in place, which, combined with the support of the wall can help to further facilitate muscular relaxation.

If would like to cover up with a blanket or equivalent, you can place it over your upper body and tuck it under your arms, so that it hugs your arms close into your body (a little like swaddling), and you feel snug and secure. Remember, you can wear socks in this or any of your restorative poses to keep your feet warm too.

Alternatively, you can fold a blanket in a long rectangular shape and place it over your abdomen to provide some light weight to this area. As an option here you can also gently tuck the sides of the blanket into your hips to create a sense of the blanket gently hugging your hips. If you have an extra pillow or cushion to hand you may wish to place it on top of the blanket on your abdomen. Allow your arms and hands to rest where it feels most comfortable for you.

Another way to use a blanket here, again, folded in a long rectangular shape, is to drape it over the soles of your feet. This will add some gentle weight to the feet and legs, as well as helping to keep your feet warm.

If you would like to cover your eyes, place a soft scarf, sleep mask or eye pillow over them.

If you start to experience a tingling sensation in your feet during this or any of the following variations of Legs up the wall – and for some of us this can occur after around five minutes – it's not a bad thing, but you can use this as your cue to carefully exit the pose as instructed above.

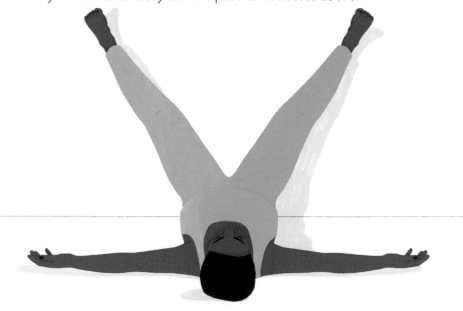

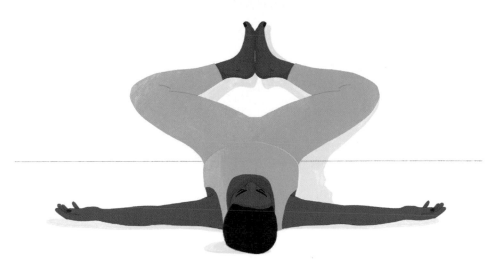

For the wide angle variation, from Legs up the wall move your legs apart as far as your hips will comfortably allow.

For the bound angle variation, from Legs up the wall bring the soles of your feet together, creating a diamond shape with your legs, and slide the outside edges of your feet down the wall towards your hips, as far down the wall as feels comfortable.

For the feet on the wall variation, your legs will not be extended all the way up the wall. Instead, the soles of your feet rest on the wall. The contact of your feet against the wall can feel grounding. This is an option to try if the soles of your feet facing the ceiling feels too much or too exposing for you (*see If rest doesn't feel relaxing* on pp. 83–4).

Also, if this is the case for you, then let yourself be here for a shorter period of time – you can start with as little as a minute and build up from there.

Stack your pillows/cushions on top of each other next to a wall. Lie on your back and rest your lower legs on top of your pillow stack with the

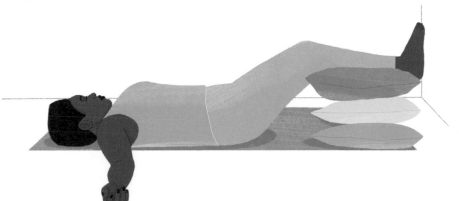

soles of your feet comfortably resting on the wall. Aim for your ankles to be in line with your knees. With this in mind, do adjust your pillow stack with more or less height if needed.

If you're using something like a dressing gown belt with no buckle, tie a knot in it to form a loop that is approximately your hip-width. Slide your feet through the loop and slide the belt up to mid-calf height. If using a belt with a buckle, use the buckle to create a loop that is approximately your hip-width and follow the above steps. The benefit of using a belt is that it will provide extra support for your legs by comfortably, yet securely, holding them in place.

Check that your chin is not pointing upwards – allow your chin to move slightly in towards your chest and place a folded blanket under your head for extra support.

If you don't wish to cover your eyes, then you could rest your soft scarf or eye pillow across your forehead to add some gentle weight.

Before settling in, you have the option to cover your body with a blanket. Alternatively, you could rest a folded blanket across your abdomen and/or a folded blanket across the tops of your lower legs.

Allow your arms and hands to rest where they feel most comfortable.

When you feel ready to move out of this pose, gently rest the soles of your feet on your pillow stack or hug your knees in towards your chest. If hugging your knees in to your chest, you may wish to gently rock from side to side a few times. This rocking movement gently massages the lower back. Carefully roll over to rest on one side. Pause here for a few breaths before gently guiding yourself up to a comfortable sitting position.

For the legs on a chair variation, in general the same principles apply.

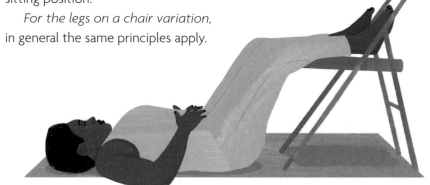

For extra comfort and ease, place a blanket or equivalent on the floor where your back and sacrum (back of the pelvis) will be resting. Have a cushion or pillow within your reach for head support.

If the chair seat (where your lower legs will be resting) has a hard surface, you may wish to place a folded blanket or pillow there for softness.

If you're using a belt, follow the steps in Legs up the wall. With Legs on a sofa/chair, placing a belt at around the mid-calf position often works better, but please do what feels best for your body.

Sit alongside your chair or sofa and carefully swing your lower legs up on to the chair seat.

Adjust the position of your hips so that your thighs form approximately a 35- to 45-degree angle from your chair/sofa. In this pose, this position with the legs is usually more comfortable for the lower back than the thighs and upper body, forming a 90-degree angle or capital L shape.

Place a cushion or pillow under your head for support

If you would like to cover up with a blanket or equivalent, try any of the options suggested for Legs up the wall. Instead of resting a folded blanket on the soles of the feet, you might like to try resting it over your lower legs, with the added option of placing a pillow on top.

When you feel ready to transition out of this pose, carefully bring the soles of your feet flat on to the edge of your sofa/chair seat or hug your knees into your chest and gently rock from side to side a few times. Pause here for a few breaths before carefully rolling over to one side to rest there. When you feel ready, carefully guide yourself up to a comfortable sitting position.

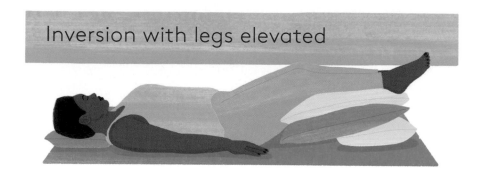

Inversion with legs elevated

···

DURATION: 2 to 5 minutes
SUGGESTED PROPS: One to three pillows, one to three cushions, one or two blankets, one soft scarf or eye mask (optional: one belt)

···

HOW TO GET THERE: For when you want something even more gentle or do not have access to a wall or chair, this pose is somewhere between Legs up the wall and Legs on a chair/sofa.

Create an incline with one or two bed pillows and a cushion by placing a cushion underneath one of the short ends of your pillow(s) so that one end is higher than the other. The higher end is where your feet will rest when you lie down.

Sit in front of your pillow/cushion incline with the higher end furthest away from you.

Slide your hips up to the lower end of your pillow/cushion incline and rest your legs on your props. Your feet should be at the higher end of the incline. If your feet are draping over the end, slide back until the backs of your heels are supported on your props.

Lie down flat on your back so that your head is below the height of your legs and feet. Note whether you would benefit from support under your head. If you find your chin is pointing up towards the ceiling, then placing a cushion, pillow or folded blanket under the head will bring the chin slightly in towards the chest, which is usually more soothing.

If you're using a belt, follow the steps in Legs up the wall and Legs on a sofa/chair.

If you're covering your body, use a blanket or equivalent to cover up.

If you would like to cover your eyes, place a soft scarf, sleep mask or eye pillow over your eyes.

When you feel ready to transition out of this pose, carefully rest the soles of your feet on your pillow/cushion incline or hug your knees into your chest (with the option to gently rock from side to side a few times). Gently roll over to rest on one side and rest here for a few breaths before guiding yourself up to a comfortable sitting position.

Supported seated forward bend

DURATION: 2 to 5 minutes
SUGGESTED PROPS: One to three pillows, one or two cushions, one or two blankets or one or two bath towels – roll a blanket or towel into a long sausage shape (optional: access to a wall, a chair, a belt or resistance band)

HOW TO GET THERE: Place a cushion or folded blanket on the surface where you will be sitting. If you feel you would benefit from support behind you, place your cushion or folded blanket next to a wall. Alternatively, you might like to rest your heels and the soles of your feet on the wall – this can feel grounding. If so, position your cushion/folded blanket so that your feet will touch the wall when you're seated.

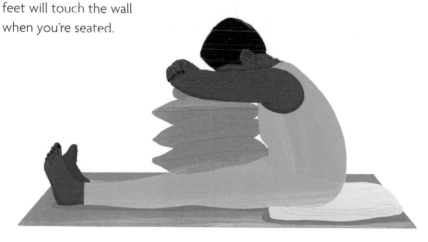

Sit on the edge (or corner) of your cushion or blanket with your legs extended in front of you. Do add extra support under your hips if you need to. If your hamstrings feel particularly tight or you feel an uncomfortable pulling sensation at the backs of your knees, place your blanket/towel roll behind your knees.

If you feel that your legs would benefit from extra support, with your legs at approximately hip-width apart, place a belt or a resistance band around your legs at mid-calf or mid-thigh level, whichever feels most comfortable for you.

Stack your pillows on top of each other and rest them on your legs. Rest your upper body on your pillows. Add a cushion on top of your pillows if you would like extra height. You could also rest your forearms on top of each other on your pillows to support your forehead. Allow your chin to tuck slightly in towards your chest to help lengthen the back of your neck.

If you would like to cover up, you can wrap a folded blanket or bath towel around your lower back and hips or drape an open blanket over the back of your body.

Allow your eyes to close or soften your gaze to a single spot so that the muscles around your eyes are able to relax.

With each exhale, visualise your physical body, softening a little more into your forward bend. Visualise any unwanted tightness or tension releasing.

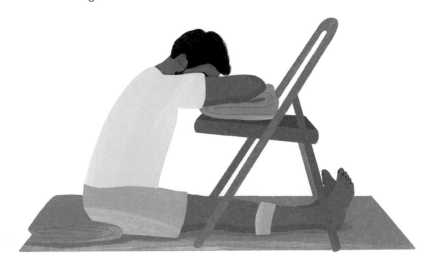

Ideally your forehead will be supported by your props. If the above option doesn't feel right for your body, you can bring the floor up to your forehead with the aid of a chair.

If using a chair, it will need to be a chair that allows you to slide your legs through it.

Place a cushion or folded blanket on the surface where you will be sitting.

Sit on the edge (or corner) of your cushion or blanket with your legs extended in front of you. If your hamstrings feel particularly tight or you feel an uncomfortable pulling sensation at the backs of your knees, place your blanket/towel roll behind the knees.

Place the chair over your legs so that the chair seat is facing your torso. If you would like to add padding to the chair seat (as this is where your forehead will be resting), place a pillow or folded blanket on to the chair seat.

Bring your upper body forward until you can rest your forearms and forehead on the chair seat. You might need to move the chair closer or further away to accommodate the proportions of your body and to ensure that you are bending forward without strain. Remember, you can elevate the hips further by sitting on an extra cushion or blanket if this feels more comfortable for your forward bend.

You can choose to elevate your forehead higher by stacking your forearms on each other on the chair seat and resting your forehead on top.

If you would like to cover up, you can wrap a folded blanket or bath towel around your lower back and hips, or drape an open blanket over the back of your body

Allow your eyes to close or soften your gaze to a single spot so that the muscles around your eyes are able to relax.

When you feel ready to exit your Supported seated forward bend, if your eyes are closed, keep them closed. Slowly lift your head and guide yourself up to sitting tall. Cup your palms over your closed eyes, blink them open and slowly remove your hands. Pause here for a several breaths before moving on.

Supported seated wide angle pose

DURATION: 2 to 5 minutes
SUGGESTED PROPS: Two or three bed pillows, two or three cushions, one or two folded blankets (optional: a chair)

HOW TO GET THERE: Place a cushion or folded blanket on to the surface where you will be sitting.

Sit on the edge (or corner) of your cushion or folded blanket and take your legs apart – as wide as feels comfortable for your hips. Add extra support under your hips if you need to. If your hamstrings feel particularly tight or you feel an uncomfortable pulling sensation at the backs of your knees, place your blanket/towel roll behind them.

Stack your pillows on top of each other and rest them lengthways in front of you. If you would like to add some height, place a cushion or two under the end of the pillows that is furthest away from you to create an incline – your head will be resting at the higher end of your incline.

Rest your body on the pillows/cushion(s) in front of you. Rest your forearms along either side of your pillows, one ear resting down on your support, allowing your chin to tuck slightly in towards your chest. Alternatively, stack your forearms on your pillows and rest your forehead on top, or one ear down on your forearms, again allowing your chin to tuck

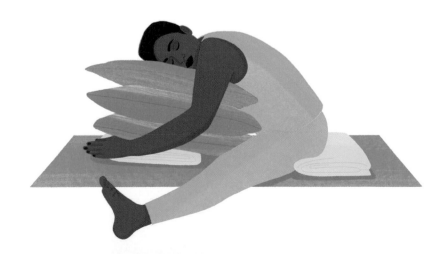

slightly in towards your chest. If you're resting one ear down, remember to turn your head to the other side while you're in this pose.

If using a chair, place a cushion or folded blanket on to the surface where you will be sitting.

Sit on the edge (or corner) of your cushion or folded blanket and take your legs apart – as wide as feels comfortable for your hips. If your hamstrings feel particularly tight or you feel an uncomfortable pulling sensation at the backs of your knees, place your blanket/towel roll behind them.

Place the chair in front of you so that the chair seat is facing your torso. If you would like to add padding to the chair seat (as this is where your forehead will be resting), place a pillow or folded blanket on to the chair seat.

Bring your upper body forward until you can rest your forearms and forehead on the chair seat. You might need to move the chair closer to you or further away to accommodate the proportions of your body and to ensure that you are bending forward without strain. You can choose to elevate your forehead higher by stacking your forearms on to each other on the chair seat and resting your forehead on top.

If you would like to cover up, you can wrap a folded blanket or bath towel around your lower back and hips, or drape an open blanket over the back of your body.

Allow your eyes to close or soften your gaze to a single spot so that the muscles around your eyes are able to relax.

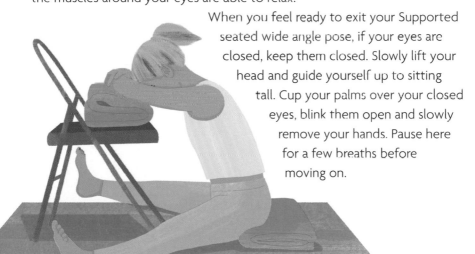

When you feel ready to exit your Supported seated wide angle pose, if your eyes are closed, keep them closed. Slowly lift your head and guide yourself up to sitting tall. Cup your palms over your closed eyes, blink them open and slowly remove your hands. Pause here for a few breaths before moving on.

Restorative rescue
– the rest sessions

In the following sections you will find a number of restorative poses and sequences you can turn to in times when you feel in need of some restorative rescue. Please feel free to dip in and out of these as much or as little as you like. I have offered various prop suggestions. However, you can also improvise with whatever items you have to hand and use more or less propping if you wish. The main thing is that you are as comfortable as possible and make these practices your own.

A note on timings

I have suggested durations for each of the poses in the sequences that follow. However, being prescriptive about how long you should spend in each pose could be stress-inducing, which would defeat the object entirely, so make this process as simple as possible for you.

If you're using an app timer, then one option would be to set intervals. For example, if you have 30 minutes to practise your sequence, you could set intervals of five minutes so that each time your timer chimes it will indicate that it's time for you to change your position or move on to the next pose.

However, if you would prefer not to do this, then an alternative approach is to stay in each pose for as long as intuitively feels right for you before moving on to the next one. If you know that you have an allotted amount of time in your day to practise your pose or sequence, say 20 minutes, you can still set a timer for that duration and know that when it chimes it will be time to bring your practice to a close.

Whichever approach you choose, what is important is that it is easy for you. There is no one right way – please go with what feels best for you.

Post-practice reflection

At the end of each practice, I have offered a question for you to reflect on. This is totally optional. However, if journaling does appeal to you, then you may find that the act of writing is helpful for processing your thoughts. Getting them out of your head and on to the page can be a way of uncluttering your mind and moving away from rumination.

Something that can also be beneficial, and something I have personally done since childhood, is free-writing (it wasn't until I discovered *The Artist's Way* by Julia Cameron as an adult that I realised this was a thing). To free-write, with a pen and paper simply allow yourself to write uncensored. Don't worry about grammar or trying to write beautiful prose – let whatever is in your head come out on to the page. Maybe a drawing or doodle will come out instead of words. For both the post-practice reflection and free-writing, I'd suggest allowing yourself a two- to five-minute time limit so that you avoid any feelings of pressure to write a certain amount. That said, if you find yourself wanting to write for longer, then please do.

Rest session for **fatigue**

Fatigue can feel as though you're carrying an extra weight around that you just can't shift. Allow your physical body to be supported by your props, so that you don't need to hold yourself up.

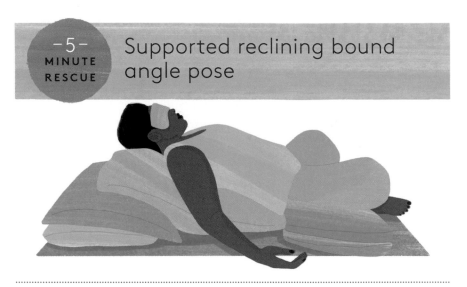

– 5 –
MINUTE
RESCUE

Supported reclining bound angle pose

DURATION: 5 to 10 minutes (up to 20 minutes is OK if you have more time) with optional psychic alternate nostril breathing (see *Breathing practices* in the *CALM* section)

SUGGESTED PROPS: One to three pillows, one to three cushions, one or two blankets, one soft scarf or eye mask

See pp. 48–9 for full instructions.

If you are using music or background sound, turn this on first. Then set your timer if you're using one.

Make any adjustments you need to before settling in to rest here until your timer lets you know that your practice has come to an end.

Sequence for fatigue

For this sequence you will only need one prop set-up for all of the poses: pillows/cushion on an incline, as described for setting up Supported reclining bound angle (*see* pp. 48–9). When moving between the poses, take your time. For the benefit of the nervous system, the transitions between the poses are as important as the poses themselves.

1 **Supported reclining bound angle pose** (5 to 20 minutes)
   See pp. 48–9 for full instructions.
2 **Supported reclining twist – version A**
   (2 to 5 minutes)
   – Keeping the knees bent, bring both knees over to your right side and allow your right hip to rest at the lower end of your pillow/cushion incline. Place a cushion between your knees.
   – Turn your torso to your right and place your hands on either side of your pillow/cushion incline before lowering your torso on to your pillow/cushion incline with your head at the higher end.
   See pp. 49–50 for full instructions.
   – Allow yourself to be here in your Supported reclining twist for up to five minutes. When you're ready to transition, carefully slide your hands back towards you along either side of your pillow(s) and press your palms down so that you can carefully lift your torso up from your props.
   – Repeat your Supported reclining twist on the other side for the same duration.
3 **Supported fish pose** (2 to 10 minutes)
   – From your Supported reclining twist, sit with your tailbone at the lower end of pillow/cushion set-up to come into supported fish pose.
   See pp. 61–3 for full instructions.
   – Rest here for between 2 and 10 minutes.
   – When you are ready to transition from Supported fish pose, bend your knees and bring the soles of your feet on to the surface you are

resting on, place your palms by your hips and press them firmly down to help you come up to sitting without needing to twist on your way up.

4 **Inversion with legs elevated** (2 to 5 minutes)
— Turn around so that you're now sitting with your pillow/cushion incline in front of you. The higher end, where your head was resting, will be furthest away from you.
See pp. 72–3 for full instructions.
— Rest here for between 2 and 5 minutes.
— To transition from your inversion, carefully place the soles of your feet on the ground on either side of your pillow incline or hug your knees into your chest.

5 **Savasana – final relaxation** (2 to 20 minutes)
— Slide your pillow(s) under the backs of your knees. Here you can either extend your legs out straight or bring the soles of the feet together into a bound angle position, supported by your pillow(s). If you intend to rest in the first position for more than 10 minutes, you may wish to place a rolled-up towel or blanket under the ankles (*see Supported restorative savasana* on pp. 34–5). Notice if you would like to adjust or add support under your head and neck.
— If you are covering your body, use a blanket or equivalent to cover up.
— If you would like to cover your eyes, place a soft scarf, sleep mask or eye pillow over your eyes.
— Rest here for between 2 and 20 minutes.
— When you're ready to close your practice, carefully bring the soles of your feet to your pillow(s) or hug your knees to your chest for a few breaths. Notice whether your body wants a stretch, a yawn or a sigh. Roll over to rest on one side, resting your head on your hands or on the backs of your arms. Carefully guide yourself up to sitting – your eyes can be closed or open – and take a few deep breaths here, thanking yourself for giving you this time. If your eyes are closed, gently open them, re-orienting yourself to the space you're in.

Post-practice reflection: What can I do to support my mind and body today? This week?

IF REST DOESN'T FEEL RELAXING

For many of us, long restorative holds can be deeply relaxing, but for some being still for extended periods and entering the pratyahara state (*see* p. 31) can result in a feeling of discombobulation or distress, because they've lost their proprioception or awareness of their physical body in time and space. When receptors in our skin, joints, muscle tissues and fascia known as proprioceptors are stimulated, our brain receives information about our body position and our body's movements, but no movement and therefore no information can be disorientating for some people. Related to this, while the physical body is still the mind can become, or at least appear to be, more active. With no distractions, any thoughts or emotions you have been suppressing can race to the surface.

However, this doesn't mean that you can't practise restorative yoga. In fact, when you're going through a tough time, feeling anxious or experiencing chronic stress, restorative practices can be particularly beneficial. In the case of a racing mind or anxiety, relaxation helps to reduce physical tension, which can then enable you to control your reactions. That said, we are all individuals and it's important to note that you might need to engage in a more active practice to help you relax. There are things you can do to adapt and tailor your practice to your needs, but it is important to do what feels right for you. Here are some suggestions to consider.

Add movement to ease yourself in: Before you begin your restorative yoga practice, incorporate movements like Cat cow flow, Seated spinal rotations or twists (*see Move your energy* on pp. 23–30 for guidance).

Progressive muscle relaxation: This involves tensing muscle groups in your body and then relaxing them. You may find doing this before you settle into a restorative pose helps to facilitate relaxation (*see Tense and release* on pp. 30–1 for guidance on how to practise this).

Shorter holds in the pose: Whatever pose or poses you would like to practise, you can start with as little as a minute or eight breaths in a posture.

Keep your eyes open: Instead of covering your eyes, soften your gaze to something in your eyeline. Softening your gaze will allow the muscles around your eyes to be relaxed.

Add weight to your body: This can be covering up with a blanket, resting folded blankets on your body or wrapping parts of your body with a blanket, as though tucking yourself in, to create a sensation of being held. This can also provide proprioceptive input (see the *Rest session for anxiety* and *Rest session for depression* for more on weighting).

Ground the soles of your feet: Allowing the soles of your feet to be in contact with a surface like a wall, the base of a sofa or hardback books can create more of a sense of feeling grounded. Having the soles of your feet on a wall in a variation of the Legs up the wall pose, for instance, can provide a feeling of standing on solid ground even though the body is supine (*see* pp. 69–70).

Add mindful movement during your practice: If it feels good and safe for you to do so, incorporate some gentle mindful movement while you are in the pose. This could be done as a way in to help you settle or as needed while you are there. For instance, depending on the pose you're in, this movement could be gently circling your wrists or ankles one way and then the other, gently turning your head to one side then the other, or turning the palms down and up. This can also be done while linking your breath to the movement – for example, inhaling as you turn your palms up and exhaling as you turn your palms down.

Kindness begins with you: Above all, kindness towards yourself, compassion for yourself, is key. Your practice is not a competition. There is no one right way. What feels right for you can vary from day to day. The berating voice inside your head is not the truth. Think of how you would treat someone who you care for deeply and offer yourself that same care.

Rest session for **anxiety**

When it comes to anxiety we often think about mental agitation. However, anxiety can be experienced in many ways and the symptoms can be physical as well as mental – for instance, unexplained muscle aches and pains, tingling skin or gastrointestinal issues.

According to the Anxiety and Depression Association of America, generalised anxiety disorder (GAD) affects 6.8 million adults, with women twice as likely to be affected as men. Related to this, it is possible to experience anxiety and depression at the same time. In her book *Yoga for Emotional Balance*, Bo Forbes brilliantly explains that our bodies can be depressed or anxious as well as our minds, and that it is possible to find ourselves in the space of simultaneously experiencing an anxious mind and depressed body, or a depressed body and anxious mind.

The following sequence addresses an approach for anxiety featuring face-down poses with the option to place some gentle weight on the body to encourage calm and grounding (if you've ever used weighted blankets you may have heard of this before). Later in this book there is a sequence relating to depression. If you do find yourself in the place of experiencing both, then I will offer some suggestions for this too. As mentioned at the start of this book, yoga is not a 'cure-all' and we are all individuals, so different things will work for each of us, but it can certainly be of help alongside other interventions and on its own when practised consistently.

ANXIOUS BODY/DEPRESSED MIND OR DEPRESSED BODY/ANXIOUS MIND

Anxious body and depressed mind – see *Rest session for anxiety* and practise with 1:1 breathing (sama vritti – inhale same length as exhale).

Depressed body and anxious mind – see *Rest session for depression* and practise with 1:2 breathing (extending your exhale).

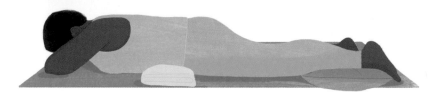

Face-down relaxation pose

....

DURATION: 5 to 10 minutes with optional diaphragmatic breathing
(see *Breathing practices* in the *CALM* section)
SUGGESTED PROPS: One or two pillows, one or two blankets, one soft
scarf or eye mask

....

Face-down relaxation pose can be practised prop-free or for extra comfort
you can practise this with the addition of blankets and pillows.

See pp. 57–8 for full instructions.

If you're using music or background sound, turn this on first. Then set
your timer. Make any adjustments you need to before settling in to rest
until your timer lets you know that your practice has come to an end.

When you feel ready to transition out of this pose, slowly slide your
hands alongside your shoulders, press your palms down on to the surface
you are resting on and bring your hips back towards your heels. Pause here
then carefully guide yourself up to a comfortable kneeling or sitting position.
Stay here for several breaths before moving on.

Sequence for anxiety

SUGGESTED PROPS: One or two cushions, one or two bed pillows, one to three blankets, one soft scarf or eye mask (optional: a chair, a bath towel)

Breath awareness: 1:2 breathing – exhalation longer than inhalation

1 **Face-down relaxation pose** (5 to 10 minutes)
   – As above.
   See pp. 57–8 for full instructions.

2 **Supported child's pose – version A or B** (2 to 5 minutes)
   – Start from your kneeling position. If you feel that your knees would benefit from some padding, place a folded blanket under them.
   See pp. 52–3 for full instructions.

3 **Side-lying relaxation pose** (2 to 20 minutes)
   See pp. 36–7 for full instructions.
   – When you're ready to close your practice, notice if your body wants a stretch or a yawn, a sigh or any other movement that feels good for you. Carefully guide yourself up to sitting – your eyes can be closed or open – and take a few deep breaths, thanking yourself for giving you this time. If your eyes are closed, gently open them, taking in your surroundings.

Post-practice reflection: I can let go of ...

Rest session for **depression**

Depression does not discriminate – any of us can experience it any stage of our lives. According to the World Health Organization, depression affects more than 264 million people of all ages globally, with more women affected than men. Depression expresses itself in a wide range of ways and can (though not always) be accompanied by feelings of anxiety. It is often characterised by low mood, but just a few of the numerous ways it can show up are physical numbness, lethargy, no longer being interested in things that used to bring you joy, deep sadness and even aggression and irritability. You may have heard the expression, 'depression is anger turned inward'. According to a 2013 study in the UK, this anger turned inward may be a contributory factor to the severity of depression.

Because there are so many signs and symptoms, and the degree to which each person experiences depression varies so much, as with anxiety, there is no 'one-size-fits-all' approach. If you are in a place where you have been experiencing depressive feelings for a long time, it is crucial to reach out, whether that starts with talking to a trusted person in your life (this could be messaging or writing to them if talking feels too hard), contacting your doctor or an organisation such as the Samaritans. If you're based in the UK, Depression UK has lots of useful links and guidance on where to find help.

The following sequence aims to re-energise by focusing on poses that create a sense of opening the front of the body with gentle back-bending – the opposite of the face-down postures in the anxiety sequence.

As with the *Rest session for anxiety* sequence, you may wish to experiment with weighting some of your restorative poses to see whether this feels soothing for you. Remember that if you don't like the addition of weight in any of the poses, you can remove it.

Supported bridge pose or Supported fish pose

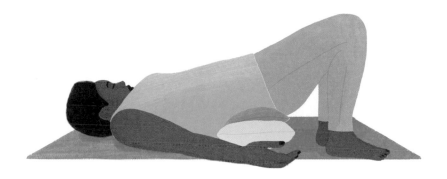

DURATION: 2 to 5 minutes

SUGGESTED PROPS: One or two pillows, one cushion, one or two blankets or four blankets (three folded, one to cover up), one cushion, one soft scarf or eye mask (optional: a belt)

Breath awareness: 1:1 breathing (sama vritti) – even inhalation and exhalation.

Supported bridge pose

See pp. 64–5 for full instructions.

While you're in supported bridge pose, remember you have the option to add some gentle weight to the body by resting a folded blanket across your abdomen or open your blanket to cover up your body.

Supported fish pose – version A

See p. 61 for full instructions.

This alternative backbend will create more of an open feeling in the front of your body.

If you're covering your body, use a blanket or equivalent to cover up. Alternatively, rest a folded blanket over your abdomen.

Rest here for between 2 and 10 minutes.

Sequence for depression

SUGGESTED PROPS: One to three pillows, one to three cushions, one to four blankets, access to a wall, chair or sofa, one soft scarf or eye mask (optional: a belt)

Breath awareness: 1:1 breathing (sama vritti) – even inhalation and exhalation

1 **Supported bridge pose or supported fish pose – version A**
   (2 to 5 minutes) As above.
   – With the option to add weight to the abdomen or legs.
2 **Legs up the wall** (2 to 10 minutes)
   – With the option to add weight to your feet or abdomen.
   See pp. 66–71 for full instructions
   – Alternatively, you can practise Legs on a chair/sofa (*see pp. 70–1*) with optional weight on legs/feet and/or optional weight on abdomen.
3 **Supported reclining bound angle pose** (2 to 10 minutes)
   – With the option to add weight to abdomen.
   See pp. 48–9 for full instructions
4 **Supported reclining pose** (2 to 20 minutes)
   See p. 38 for full instructions
   – With the option to add weight on to your body.
   Or **Supported restorative savasana** (5 to 20 minutes)
   See pp. 34–5 for full instructions
   – With the option to add weight on to your body.
   – When you feel ready to close your practice, roll over so that you're lying on your side. From here, guide yourself up to a comfortable sitting position. Thank yourself for devoting this time for your practice.

Post-practice reflection: When is the last time I did something nice for myself? What nice thing can I do for myself today? This week?

Rest session for **grief**

There is a saying that, 'Grief is love with nowhere to go'. That felt very apt to me when my mother, who I love dearly and was incredibly close to, passed away unexpectedly. The very practices I am sharing with you in this book are the ones that I turned to, especially in those very early stages of grief, which happened to coincide with the arrival of Covid-19 in the UK where I live.

But grief is not only caused by the loss of close loved ones. Many of us experience the deep sorrow and pain of grief for a whole host of reasons. The emergence of Covid and the impact it has had on our lives has resulted in a collective grief as well as personal. These are also practices I turned to after the 2020 death of George Floyd and to process the reality (and yet another reminder) that in the minds of far too many, Black Lives – lives like mine – still do not Matter. In her book, *Restorative Yoga for Ethnic and Race-Based Stress and Trauma*, Dr Gail Parker writes about the potential of restorative yoga to alleviate some of the suffering and distress people experience as a result of ethnic and race-based stress and trauma (which is distinct from PTSD). There is not a 'life hack' for grief and it is not linear, but wherever your grief is stemming from, know that there is and will be a way through. Give yourself permission to grieve fully. This practice may be of help in those times.

Legs up the wall or Legs on a sofa/chair

DURATION: 2 to 10 minutes
SUGGESTED PROPS: A wall (or sofa or chair), one cushion, one or two pillows, one to three blankets, one soft scarf or eye mask (optional: a belt)

If you are using music or background sound, turn this on first. Then set your timer.

Legs up the wall (2 to 10 minutes)

You can practise using just the wall or (I'd recommend) with the addition of props for extra support. Use as many props as you need to.

See pp. 66–71 for full instructions.

Legs on a sofa/chair (2 to 10 minutes)

See pp. 70–1 for full instructions.

Both these poses are inversions (the feet are raised above the heart and head), but if for any reason you do not wish to invert – for instance, if you are currently menstruating (*see* p. 96) – then you could practice *Supported reclining pose* for 2 to 20 minutes (*see p. 38 for instructions*) or *Supported reclining bound angle pose* (*see pp. 48–9 for instructions*) instead, with optional weight on the abdomen in the form of a folded blanket and/or pillow for either pose.

Sequence for grief

SUGGESTED PROPS: A wall (or sofa or chair), one to three cushions, one to three pillows, one to three blankets, one soft scarf or eye mask (optional: a belt)

1 **Supported reclining pose** (2 to 20 minutes)
   See p. 38 for full instructions.
   – Or **Supported reclining bound angle pose** (2 to 20 minutes)
   See pp. 48–9 for full instructions

2 **Supported reclining twist – version A** (2 to 5 minutes on each side)
   – With the same prop set-up (pillow/cushion incline) as the previous pose.
   See pp. 49–50 for full instructions

3 **Supported child's pose** (2 to 5 minutes)
   See pp. 52–3 for full instructions
   – OR **Face-down relaxation pose** (5 to 10 minutes)
   See pp. 57–8 for full instructions.

4 **Legs up the wall or legs on a sofa/chair** (2 to 10 minutes) with optional weight on legs/feet and/or optional weight on abdomen.
   See pp. 66–71 for full instructions.

5 **Side-lying relaxation pose** (5 to 20 minutes)
   See pp. 36–7 for full instructions
   – Or **Supported restorative savasana** (5 to 20 minutes)
   See pp. 34–5 for full instructions
   – With the option of a blanket over abdomen and chest.

Post-practice reflection: How can I take care of myself in the moments when grief feels overwhelming? What support systems do I have available to help me?

Part One: Rest

Rest session for **PMS**

Premenstrual syndrome (PMS) is the term for the symptoms that can be experienced in the weeks before menstruation. Though the number of symptoms and their severity vary from person to person and from month to month, common ones include bloating, mood swings, feeling anxious or irritable, tiredness or difficulty sleeping. According to the NHS it is not known precisely why PMS occurs, although changes in hormone levels during the menstrual cycle are thought to be a factor. It is understood that reducing stress can be helpful for PMS, which is why, along with its capacity to aid symptoms such as anxiety and insomnia, restorative yoga can be beneficial at this time (*see also Rest session for anxiety* and *Rest session for insomnia*). The following is a practice that may be of help in the weeks and days before your period starts.

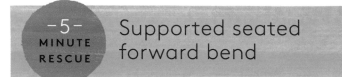

–5–
MINUTE
RESCUE

Supported seated forward bend

DURATION: 2 to 5 minutes
SUGGESTED PROPS: One to three pillows, one or two cushions, one or two blankets or one or two bath towels — roll a blanket or towel into a long sausage shape (optional: access to a wall, a chair, a belt)

See pp. 73–5 for full instructions.

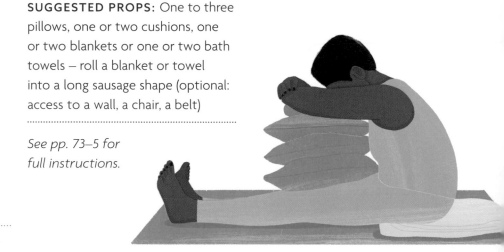

▶ **WHEN YOU HAVE MORE TIME**
Sequence for PMS

SUGGESTED PROPS: One to three pillows, one or two cushions, one or two blankets or one or two bath towels – roll a blanket or towel into a long sausage shape (optional: access to a wall, a chair, a belt)

1 **Supported seated forward bend** (2 to 5 minutes)
   As above.
   See pp. 73–5 for full instructions.
2 **Supported bound angle pose** (1 to 3 minutes)
   See pp. 42 3 for full instructions.
3 **Supported seated wide angle pose** (2 to 5 minutes)
   See pp 76–7 for full instructions.
4 **Supported bridge pose** (2 to 5 minutes)
   See pp. 64–5 for full instructions.
   – After exiting your Supported bridge pose, let the backs of your knees rest on your pillow(s)/blanket(s). You can choose to stay here for Supported restorative savasana or transition to Face-down relaxation pose.
5 **Supported restorative savasana** (2 to 20 minutes)
   See pp. 34–5 for full instructions.
   – Or **Face-down relaxation pose** (2 to 20 minutes)
   See pp. 57–8 for instructions.

Post-practice reflection: What situations or people have caused you stress recently? How can you give yourself space from these situations or people?

PRACTISING INVERSIONS DURING MENSTRUATION

In yoga, an inversion is a pose that takes you upside down, usually defined as when the head is below the heart or the hips are higher than the head. When I first began to practise yoga, I learned that inversions should be avoided during menstruation. This is because, energetically speaking, apana (the downward flow of energy) is disrupted by taking the body – or specifically, with regard to menstruation, the uterus – upside down or above the head. This is what has been taught via B.K.S. Iyengar's school of yoga and given that this is where restorative yoga was developed, inversions are generally omitted from practice during menstruation. While some schools of yoga agree with this, others don't. From a biological perspective it was at one time thought that inversions may result in menstrual blood travelling in the opposite direction through the fallopian tubes (known as retrograde menstruation), providing the opportunity for uterine tissue to attach itself there and consequently increasing the risk of endometriosis. However, according to endometriosis.org, 'There is little evidence that endometrial cells can attach to women's pelvic organs and grow' and in 1984 research showed that 90 per cent of women experience retrograde menstruation while only 10 per cent of women develop endometriosis and even then a connection to retrograde menstruation is unclear. So while it appears that from a biological perspective there is no definite reason to not invert during menstruation, I have found over the years of my own practice that during my period, my body prefers to slow down and skip inverted postures. All our experiences are different and it is important to tune into what feels right for your body.

Rest session for **pregnancy**

Pregnancy can be a wonderful and exciting time and, while there is no reason to stop many of the things you did pre-pregnancy, let's not underestimate the fact that you are growing a human (in some cases, more than one at the same time!), so it's highly likely that your energy levels won't be what they were. If ever there was a time to put yourself at the top of your list, it's now. Restorative yoga can alleviate the fatigue that may occur during pregnancy due to hormonal shifts and the extra weight your body is carrying. The following sequence is designed specifically for pregnancy. However, as each pregnancy is different, before practising these poses I would recommend showing them to your doctor to ensure that they are appropriate for you.

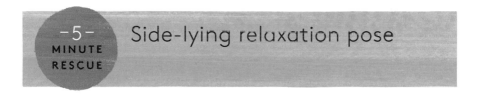

-5- **MINUTE RESCUE** Side-lying relaxation pose

DURATION: 5 to 20 minutes
SUGGESTED PROPS: One or two cushions, one or two bed pillows, one or two blankets, a soft scarf or sleep mask to cover your eyes

If you are using music or background sound, turn this on first. Set your timer. *See pp. 36–7 for full instructions.*

Lie on your left side (lying flat on the back during pregnancy is usually inadvisable after 20 weeks). In addition, you might wish to place a folded blanket or a pillow under the left side of your bump for extra support.

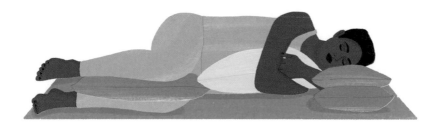

SUGGESTED PROPS: One to three cushions, one or two bed pillows, one or two blankets, one soft scarf or eye mask (optional: access to a wall)

TIP: If getting up and down from the floor poses too much of a challenge, try practising this sequence on your bed. Wherever you practise, you might wish to use extra propping – do use as many pillows or cushions as you wish to ensure that you are as comfortable as you possibly can be.

1 **Supported bound angle pose** (1 to 3 minutes)
This pose can be a helpful one to practise regularly for birth preparation as it gently opens the hips and groin.

If you feel that you would benefit from extra support for your back, you may wish to sit against a wall.

Place a cushion or folded blankets on the floor to sit on. This will elevate your hips to allow your spine to be in a neutral position (not rounding through the upper back), provide support for your sitting bones and alleviate lower back discomfort.

Bring the soles of your feet together so that your knees form a diamond shape with your legs. Place cushions (or equivalent) under each leg. If you have been experiencing any knee discomfort, add support here and move the feet further forward.

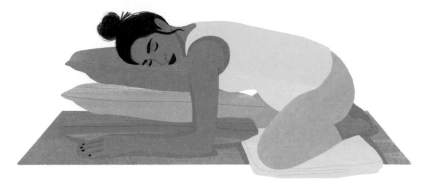

2 Modified supported child's pose (1 to 5 minutes)

This is similar to Supported child's pose, but with extra propping.

SUGGESTED PROPS: Two or three pillows, two or three blankets (or equivalent), one or two cushions, one bath towel (rolled into a long sausage shape), one soft scarf or eye mask

If you're practising on the floor rather than a bed, you also have the option to practise the variation of Supported child's pose with a chair (see Supported child's pose – version B on p. 54 for instructions). If practising the chair variation, allow space for your bump so that there is no compression of your abdomen.

If you would like padding for your knees, place a folded blanket on to the surface where your knees will be resting.

Place two or three pillows stacked on top of each other lengthways in front of you. If you would prefer to create an incline so that your head is elevated higher, then you can place a cushion at the end of the pillows that is furthest away from you.

From your kneeling position, adjust your knees so that they are wider than hip-width.

Carefully lower your upper body down on to your pillow(s) so that there is space for your bump and no compression of your abdomen.

Position your arms comfortably; here are two options:

• Place one forearm on top of the other on your pillows and rest your forehead there. If you would like padding, you could place a soft scarf or eye pillow on top of your hands.

• Place your forearms along either side of your pillows and rest one ear down on to your pillows. Allow your chin to tuck slightly in towards your chest so that the back of your neck is lengthened. When you feel ready, turn your head so that your opposite ear can rest on your pillows. This will also mean that both sides of the neck (the large sternocleidomastoid muscles that often feel tense and sore) receive a gentle stretch.

If this modified Supported child's pose feels too low, then you could try Supported child's pose with a chair (see version B on p. 54) instead. If neither version works because being on your knees is uncomfortable, then you could try this Modified face-down relaxation pose. In this variation, we make sure your bump is not touching the floor or the surface you're resting on:

2a Modified face-down relaxation pose (1 to 5 minutes)

SUGGESTED PROPS: Two to four pillows, two or three blankets, one to three cushions, one bath towel (rolled into a long sausage shape), one soft scarf or eye mask

Place a blanket on to the surface that you will be resting on so that there will be softness under your knees and lower legs.

In front of you, place two to three pillows stacked on top of each other lengthways.

Between the pillows and your body place another pillow – this could be placed on top of two cushions placed alongside each other for extra height. If propped high enough, your knees will be elevated, which will further take away any unwanted pressure from the knees. Lie forward with this pillow at your hip crease and with your bump resting over the

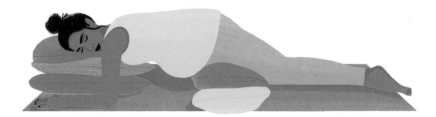

edge. If your lower legs feel like they need support, place a rolled-up towel behind you, where your feet are. Let the tops of your feet rest on the towel so that your ankles are supported.

Rest your head and chest on to the stacked pillows in front of you with one ear resting down and your arms resting along either side of your pillows. If you feel any discomfort in your arms or shoulders, try resting your forearms along either side of your head on your pillows or place a cushion along either side of your pillows to prop your arms up.

It is very important that there is space for your bump so that there is no compression on your abdomen. Your bump will be facing down or facing the floor, but not touching it. If your bump is making contact with the floor, add some more height to your props.

Remember to turn your head to the opposite side.

When you're ready to transition from this pose, carefully slide your hands back towards you and press your palms down to ease your upper body away from your props and guide yourself to a comfortable sitting position on your pillows or cushions, so that your hips are higher than your knees. Pause here until you feel ready to move to your next pose.

3 **Side-lying relaxation with legs elevated** (5 to 15 minutes)
This pose may be of help when your legs feel heavy or swollen. It is identical to Side-lying relaxation pose, with the addition of props to elevate and support the lower legs so that there is a mild inversion.

When you feel ready to close your practice, carefully guide yourself up to a comfortable sitting position and pause here for a few breaths, noting any differences to how you now feel compared to before your practice.

Post-practice reflection: Today, being pregnant feels ...

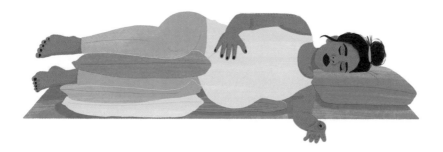

Rest session for **post-birth**

Welcoming a new baby is incredibly joyful, but those first few weeks and months can also be overwhelming and exhausting. On days when the prospect of even getting showered seems impossible, the notion of having any time for yourself can feel like a fantasy. If you are fortunate enough to have a network around you then it is important to reach out and let others support you. Just as important is having ways to support yourself. This is where restorative yoga – even just a few minutes while your baby is asleep or maybe between feeds – can be of help, not only as a way of caring for and supporting yourself (quite literally, with your props), but also for improving your energy levels during the fourth trimester.

On a physical level, a pose such as Supported reclining bound angle can help to ease the tightness in the upper back and shoulders that may occur from holding, carrying and feeding your baby, while a posture such as Supported child's pose can help to alleviate lower back tightness too. This, in turn can allow you feel more relaxed and be in a better position to care for those who need you. If you are new parents, the following sequence is designed particularly with the parent who has given birth in mind, but it is important to note that both parents can benefit from these poses.

– 5 – **MINUTE RESCUE**	Any one of the poses in the sequence for post-birth

I would recommend that you pick your favourite from the poses listed below.

If you are using music or background sound, turn this on first. Then set your timer. That said, if using a timer is unfeasible (or seems ridiculous under the circumstances!) then try to allow yourself to be in your chosen pose(s) for at least eight to 10 breaths.

Sequence for post-birth

SUGGESTED PROPS: One to three cushions, two to three bed pillows, one to three blankets, one soft scarf or eye mask (optional: a chair/sofa, a bath towel, a belt)

1 **Supported reclining bound angle pose** (5 to 20 minutes)
   See pp. 48–9 for full instructions.
2 **Supported child's pose – version A, B or C** (2 to 10 minutes)
   See pp. 52–6 for full instructions.
3 **Legs up the wall or legs on a sofa/chair** (2 to 10 minutes)
   See pp. 66–71 for full instructions.
   – If practising Legs up the wall, you can practise using just the wall or with the addition of props for extra support.
4 **Supported restorative savasana** (2 to 20 minutes)
   See pp. 34–5 for full instructions.

Post-practice reflection: Today I am proud of myself for ...

Part One: Rest

Rest session for **frazzled parents** and **caregivers**

It's easy to put yourself at the bottom of your own list when you're responsible for caring for others, whether that's caring for children, our elders, partners, vulnerable members of the community or any role that involves providing vital support. No matter how rewarding this role can be, caregiver stress is real so looking after yourself is essential. As ever, if you don't care for yourself, sooner or later you won't be able to be there for the people who rely on you. Where possible, seek out support and accept help from others. One of the gifts of restorative yoga is that the practice itself offers support. Whether you practise one or all of the poses that follow, allow your props to fully support you and hold you up.

–5–
MINUTE
RESCUE

Legs on a chair/sofa

DURATION: 2 to 10 minutes
SUGGESTED PROPS: Access to a chair or sofa, one cushion or pillow for head support, one blanket, one soft scarf or eye mask (optional: a belt)

See pp. 70–1 for full instructions.

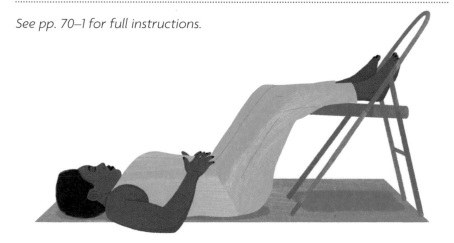

▶ WHEN YOU HAVE MORE TIME Sequence for frazzled parents and caregivers

SUGGESTED PROPS: Two to three pillows, two to three cushions, access to a chair or sofa, one or two blankets, one soft scarf or eye mask (optional: a belt)

REMINDER: You can pick just one of these poses to practise if you don't have time to do a whole sequence.

1 **Supported child's pose** (2 to 10 minutes)
   See pp. 52–3 for full instructions.

2 **Supported reclining twist – version A or B** (2 to 5 minutes on each side)
   REMINDER: Allow your abdomen to be soft. You might notice your navel gently rising and falling while you are here.
   See pp. 49–52 for full instructions.

3 **Supported reclining bound angle pose** (5 to 20 minutes)
   See pp. 48–9 for full instructions.

4 **Legs up the wall or legs on chair/sofa** (2 to 10 minutes)
   As above.
   See pp. 66–71 for full instructions.

5 **Side-lying relaxation pose** (2 to 20 minutes)
   See pp. 36–7 for full instructions.

Post-practice reflection: Where do I most need support from others?

Rest session for **perimenopause** and **menopause**

Restorative yoga is particularly effective at easing chronic stress. This is especially relevant to menopause, because we know that stress exacerbates all menopause symptoms. Menopause is reached after 12 consecutive months without a period (where there is no other reason for periods to have stopped). Typically this happens in our early fifties, so we tend to think that menopause is something we needn't concern ourselves with until then. However, perimenopause – the time leading up to menopause – is significant because as oestrogen depletes, many of the symptoms associated with menopause arise.

You might sail through this transition with total ease or you might, as is more common, experience some symptoms. Hot flushes and night sweats are the most widely known, but other, less talked-about symptoms include brain fog, anxiety, depression, new allergies, dizziness and paresthesia (sensations of tingling or numb extremities). Every experience is different and although more research is needed, it appears that your ethnicity may have a bearing on your symptoms and your age when you reach menopause. As well as nutrition, exercise and investigating whether HRT or supplements may be right for you, yoga can be helpful as we move into menopause and beyond.

−5− MINUTE RESCUE	Supported seated wide angle pose

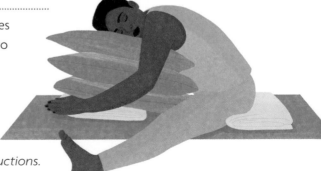

DURATION: 2 to 5 minutes
SUGGESTED PROPS: Two to three bed pillows, two to three cushions, one or two folded blankets (optional: a chair)

See pp. 76–7 for full instructions.

▶ WHEN YOU HAVE MORE TIME Sequence for perimenopause and menopause

SUGGESTED PROPS: One to three pillows, one or two cushions, one or two blankets or one or two bath towels – roll a blanket or towel into a long sausage shape (optional: access to a wall, a chair, a belt)

1 **Supported seated wide angle pose** (2 to 5 minutes)
   As above.
   See pp. 76–7 for full instructions.
2 **Supported reclining bound angle pose** (2 to 15 minutes)
   See pp. 48–9 for full instructions.
3 **Supported child's pose** (2 to 5 minutes)
   See pp. 52–3 for full instructions.
4 **Supported bridge pose** (2 to 5 minutes)
   See pp. 64–5 for full instructions.
5 **Legs up the wall** (2 to 10 minutes)
   See pp. 66–71 for full instructions.
6 **Supported restorative savasana** (2 to 20 minutes)
   See pp. 34–5 for full instructions.

Post-practice reflection: What am I ready to welcome (more of) into my life?

Rest session for **endometriosis**

Endometriosis is a condition that can affect anyone of childbearing age who has a uterus (womb). It can be debilitating and difficult to diagnose (diagnosis takes on average seven and a half years). It occurs when cells similar to those found in the lining of the uterus are found elsewhere in the body. Those cells behave in the same way as those in the uterus, reacting to the menstrual cycle. While the cells inside the uterus can leave the body as a period each month, the cells outside cannot, so when they bleed this can result in chronic pain and inflammation. Some common reported symptoms include pelvic pain, heavy and/or painful periods, difficulty conceiving, pain during or after sex, pain when going to the toilet and fatigue.

The cause of endometriosis is as yet unknown and at present there is no cure. Yoga is one of a number of lifestyle adaptions that may be of help in managing symptoms. Restorative yoga in particular can allow the tight muscles and connective tissue (which may be constricted with pain) around the abdomen and pelvis to soften. Be very kind to yourself, especially if you are experiencing a flare-up. If in doubt, do check with your doctor.

– 5 –
MINUTE RESCUE

Supported reclining bound angle pose

DURATION: 5 to 20 minutes
SUGGESTED PROPS: One to three pillows, one to three cushions, one or two blankets, one soft scarf or eye mask

See pp. 48–9 for full instructions.
If very gentle weight on the abdomen is soothing for you, consider resting a folded blanket here or a heat pack (such as a heated wheat bag) while you are in this pose.

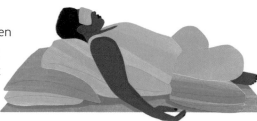

Sequence for endometriosis

SUGGESTED PROPS: Two to three pillows, two to three blankets, two to three cushions, one soft scarf or eye mask

1 **Supported reclining bound angle pose** (5 to 20 minutes)
   As above.
   See pp. 48–9 for full instructions.

2 **Supported fish pose – version B** (2 to 5 minutes)
   See pp. 62–3 for full instructions.
   – You have the option to use blankets instead – two or three folded into a long rectangular shape – if lying back over pillows feels too strong. If you are using blankets, which will be a lower height than pillows, you might find that you don't need a cushion for head support. Try with and without a cushion under your head to see what feels most comfortable for you.

3 **Supported child's pose** (2 to 5 minutes)
   – You could place a heat pack or gentle weight on your lower back or sacrum here.
   See pp. 52–3 for full instructions.

4 **Legs up the wall** (2 to 10 minutes)
   See pp. 66–71 for full instructions.
   REMINDER: You can omit this pose if you are on your period.

5 **Supported reclining pose** (2 to 20 minutes)
   See pp. 38 for full instructions.

Post-practice reflection: What are my current physical, emotional and mental needs? What steps can I take to fulfil some of these?

Rest session for **insomnia**

There are various potential causes of insomnia, whether chronic or short-term. Whatever the reason, when sleep escapes you, to say it can be draining and frustrating is an understatement. It is worth looking at your daily routine to see if there are any habits that might be contributing (*see* pp. 169–70). Formulating a wind-down routine at the end of the day may be of help too – *see Putting the day to bed* on pp. 169–72 for suggestions, including the *Bedtime pages* practice. Getting thoughts that might be keeping you up at night out of your head and on to the page before preparing to go to sleep can be especially helpful if you are prone to rumination. Here is a sequence that you can do in bed. It could be practised at bedtime or if you wake up in the night.

Rather than timings, I have offered a number of breaths as the suggested duration for each pose. This avoids using a timer (especially on a smartphone as blue light at night can worsen insomnia) and also because when trying to fall asleep, breath awareness may be of help. A few breathing options to here are 1:1 breathing (sama vritti), 1:2 breathing and psychic alternate nostril breathing (*see* pp. 127–30 in the *CALM* section).

> **–5–**
> **MINUTE**
> **RESCUE**
> ## Supported reclining bound angle pose or Legs up the wall

Supported reclining bound angle pose (16 to 32 breaths)
You can practise this pose as you normally would (*see* below), or, if you prefer using fewer props in bed, use just two pillows. Lying on your back in bed, place one pillow under your head. If necessary, squish this pillow into the sides of your neck to ensure that your head and neck feel supported. Place your second pillow behind your knees. Bring the soles of your feet together and allow your knees to fall to either side in a bound

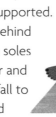

angle position. If necessary, adjust the position of the pillow at the knees to ensure that your legs and hips feel supported.

If you have three pillows, lying on your back in bed, place one pillow under your head. Again, squish this pillow into the sides of your neck. Bring the soles of your feet together and allow your knees to fall out to either side. Take your two remaining pillows and place one under each leg, positioning them to ensure that your legs and hips feel supported.

Legs up the wall (16 to 32 breaths)

If your bed is against a wall, this can be practised against the wall. If your bed is not against a wall, practise with your legs resting on the headboard.

If you have one pillow, have your pillow within reach to use for head support. Sit down on your bed with one hip alongside the wall or headboard. Carefully swing your legs and feet up on to the wall.

Alternatively, if your hamstrings feel tight, kneel as close to the wall as possible with your back facing it. Lean your upper body forward, carefully roll on to your back and swing your legs and feet up on to the wall.

For whichever approach you choose, once you have your feet (heels) touching the wall, you can choose how close the backs of your legs are to the wall. Usually, having your hips away from the wall (legs at roughly 35 to 45 degrees) is gentler and less of a stretch along the back of the body (especially hamstrings, hips and lower back). Also, this position (with your hips away from the wall) is preferable in terms of allowing the abdomen and diaphragm to soften and therefore facilitate more ease with breathing.

Having the backs of your legs and hips touching the wall (so that your body forms more of a capital L shape) will usually create more of a stretching sensation along the back of your body. With this in mind, please do adjust the position of your hips to where it feels most comfortable for you to stay for a while by either shuffling your hips closer to or further away from the wall.

When you feel ready to transition out of this pose, carefully bring the soles of your feet flat on to the wall and slide them down. Pause here for a few breaths before carefully rolling over to one side to rest there.

If you have two or three pillows, you may wish to elevate your hips slightly by placing a pillow close to the wall. You could stack two pillows on top of each other here if your pillows are thin. Have another pillow within reach for head support.

Sequence for insomnia

SUGGESTED PROPS: Two or three bed pillows

1 **Supported reclining bound angle pose** (16 to 32 breaths)
   As above.
2 **Supported half-frog pose** (8 to 16 breaths on each side)
   Roll over so that you're lying on your front. Pillows are optional.

   If you're not using pillows, place one hand on top of the other and rest one ear down on the back of your hands. Slide your right leg out to the right on your bed with your knee bent (approximately a 90-degree shape so that your right knee is level with your right hip).

   If you have one pillow, you can rest it lengthways under your torso so that your tummy, chest and head are supported. Rest one ear down on your pillow. With your arms and hands you can hug the top of the pillow or with bent elbows form a 'cactus' shape with your arms – forearms and palms resting down on your bed. Slide your right leg out to the right on your bed with your knee bent (approximately a 90-degree shape so that your right knee is level with your right hip). However, if you feel your right hip would benefit from support, place your pillow under your right leg.

   If you have two pillows, follow the steps for one pillow, placing your first pillow under your torso and your second pillow under your right leg.

   Remember to do both sides. When you're ready to swap legs, carefully slide your right leg behind you so that both legs are extended straight behind you. Gently sway your hips side to side a few times. Slide your left leg out to the left on your bed with your knee bent (approximately a ninety-degree shape so that your left knee is level with your left hip). Turn your head so that your opposite ear is resting down. Make adjustments to any pillows you are using for extra support.
3 **Supported child's pose** (8 to 16 breaths)
   From your Supported half-frog pose, with both legs straight behind you

and palms rested down on your bed alongside your shoulders, slide your hands back and hips towards your heels.

If you're not using pillows, place one forearm on top of the other and rest your forehead down on your arms. It's OK if your hips do not happen to touch your heels, but do allow your hips to move back in that direction.

If you're using two or three pillows, follow the above steps and stack two to three pillows on top of each other lengthways and rest your upper body on the pillows for support. Ensure your tummy, chest and head are supported. Rest one ear down on your pillows. With your arms and hands you can either hug your pillows or rest your forearms and palms down on your bed along either side of your pillows. If you would like some support between your thighs and calves, place one pillow between them. Remember to turn your head partway through your time in Supported child's pose so that your opposite ear is resting down.

An alternative pose is to carefully roll over on to your back and hug your knees in towards your chest (either placing your palms on your shins or on the back of each thigh)

4 **Supported reclining twist** (8 to 16 breaths on each side)
If you're using two or three pillows, carefully come to lying on your back and place a pillow under your head. Bend your knees and bring the soles of your feet to your bed. Place one or two pillows between your knees. Take your arms out to either side, palms facing up, elbows at shoulder height (either with arms straight or elbows bent so that your arms are in a 'cactus' shape). Carefully bring both knees over to the right towards the bed so that you're in a twist. Allow your legs to be in an approximately 90-degree shape so that your knees are about the same height as your hips.

5 **Legs up the wall** (16 to 32 breaths)
As above. REMINDER: You can omit this pose if you are on your period.

6 **Savasana – sleeping pose of your choice**
Choose the position you would like to fall asleep in that feels most comfortable.
Supported restorative savasana
See pp. 34–5 for instructions.
Side-lying relaxation pose
See pp. 36–7 for instructions.

Rest session for everyday **calm**

This is a restorative chair yoga sequence, an all-round, everyday sequence that brings the floor up to you rather than requiring you to get on to the floor. Feel free to practise any of the following poses individually too.

– 5 –
MINUTE
RESCUE

Supported child's pose – version C

DURATION: Up to 5 minutes
SUGGESTED PROPS: Two chairs, two to three bed pillows, two to three cushions, one or two blankets, one soft scarf or sleep mask (optional – two hardback books if you need to elevate your feet)

Have all of the props you would like to use within easy reach. Sit in one chair with the opposite chair facing you. Depending on the chair you are sitting on, you might wish to sit on a cushion or a folded blanket for extra comfort.
See pp. 55–6 for full instructions.

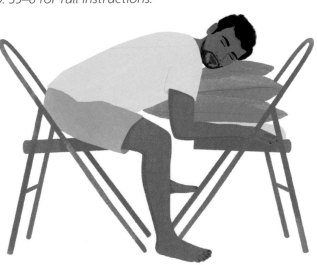

Sequence for everyday calm

SUGGESTED PROPS: Two chairs, two to three bed pillows, two to three cushions, one or two blankets, one soft scarf or eye mask (optional – two hardback books if you need to elevate your feet, a belt or resistance band)

1 **Supported child's pose – version C** (up to 5 minutes)
   As opposite.
2 **Chair-supported bound angle pose – version A or B** (up to 5 minutes)
   Remove your pillows from your second chair and place your feet on the chair seat in front of you.
   See pp. 44 7 for full instructions.
3 **Seated savasana** (up to 20 minutes)
   See p. 39 for full instructions.

Post-practice reflection: Where can I inject more joy into today? This week?

Rest session for **burnout**

Burnout is often, though not always, related to work. If you find yourself experiencing a lack of energy, cynicism and disillusionment around work, little or no satisfaction in your achievements, sleep problems, turning to food or substances to feel better or to numb out, or the emergence of physical symptoms (such as headaches or digestive issues) you may be in the midst of burnout. It is a gradual process and you might not even realise burnout is happening until you're at a very low point. Aside from addressing the root causes, setting time aside to get your body out of a stress response is important. Taking this time for yourself may also help provide clarity on your best next steps. The restorative postures can also provide support for any physical tiredness or exhaustion you might be experiencing. In addition, consider some of the practices suggested in the *CALM* section of this book, in particular *Pranayama* (pp. 126–9), *Body scanning* (pp. 146–8), *yoga nidra* (pp. 148–9) and *Boundaries* (pp. 161–8).

– 5 –
MINUTE RESCUE

Legs up the wall or Legs on a chair/sofa

DURATION: 2 to 10 minutes

Legs up the wall
See pp. 66–71 for full instructions.
Legs on a chair/sofa
See pp. 70–1 for full instructions.

Sequence for burnout

SUGGESTED PROPS: Access to a wall, sofa or chair, two to three pillows, two to three cushions, one or two blankets, one soft scarf or eye mask

1 **Legs up the wall or Legs on chair/sofa** (2 to 10 minutes)
   As above.
   See pp. 66–71 for full instructions.
2 **Supported seated wide angle pose** (2 to 5 minutes)
   See pp. 76–7 for full instructions.
3 **Supported reclining bound angle pose** (5 to 20 minutes)
   See pp. 48–9 for full instructions.
4 **Supported restorative savasana** (2 to 20 minutes)
   See pp. 34–5 for instructions.

Post-practice reflection: Where can I do less today? This week?

Rest session for **headache**

Stress is a common trigger for headaches, making restorative yoga ideally placed to help alleviate them, particularly migraines, because for some people more active practices may actually be a trigger. A 2020 study showed that migraine sufferers who practised yoga and relaxation techniques alongside medication had fewer and less intense migraine days than when using medical treatment alone. Savasana with guided yoga nidra, pranayama (breathing practices) such as alternate nostril breathing and bee breath and mudras (hand gestures) are just a few of the yoga practices that were included in this study. You will find more on *pranayama* (pp. 126–9), *mudras* (pp. 142–5) and *yoga nidra* (pp. 148–50) in the *CALM* section of this book. So if you've never tried yoga before or have found more active yoga practices unhelpful, it may be time to consider incorporating restorative yoga into your routine, especially if you know that your headaches tend to be stress-related.

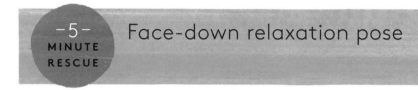

– 5 –
MINUTE
RESCUE

Face-down relaxation pose

DURATION: 5 to 20 minutes
SUGGESTED PROPS: One or two pillows, one or two blankets, one soft scarf or eye mask

See pp. 57–8 for full instructions.

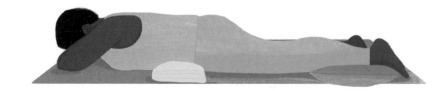

Sequence for headache

SUGGESTED PROPS: One to three pillows, two to three cushions, one or two blankets, one soft scarf or eye mask (optional: a chair)

1 **Face-down relaxation pose** (5 to 20 minutes)
   See pp. 57–8 for full instructions.
2 **Supported child's pose** (2 to 5 minutes)
   See pp. 52–3 for full instructions.
3 **Supported reclining bound angle pose** (5 to 20 minutes)
   See pp. 48–9 for full instructions.
   If a very gentle weight on the forehead is soothing for you, you can rest an eye pillow or soft scarf across your forehead, gently wrap a scarf around your forehead or rest a folded towel across your forehead.
4 **Supported seated forward bend** (2 to 5 minutes)
   See pp. 73–5 for full instructions.
5 **Supported bridge pose (option: to elevate the legs)** (2 to 5 minutes)
   See pp. 64–5 for full instructions.
   If you would like to elevate your legs, lift one foot and then the other off the ground. You can either keep your knees bent or reach your feet up towards the sky. While your feet are in the air, add some movement by circling your ankles one way and then the other or alternate between pointing your toes and flexing your feet. When you would like to lower your legs again, carefully place one foot and then the other back down.
6 **Supported restorative savasana** (2 to 20 minutes)
   See pp. 34–5 for full instructions.
   Or **Side-lying relaxation pose** (2 to 20 minutes)
   See pp. 36–7 for full instructions.

Post-practice reflection: Where in my life can I support myself better? Where can I reach out to others for support?

Rest session for **post-workout**

Be honest – how many times have you skipped your post-workout cool down or bypassed rest days? Rest is an incredibly important part of recovery, so you will be doing yourself a disservice if you don't take it as seriously as your training. Help your body (and mind) to down-regulate and repair by incorporating some restorative yoga into your routine.

When I was running regularly, I found the feeling of opening that restorative yoga provided as well as the release of muscular tension and calming of the mind invaluable. Though the feeling of a stretch may be a byproduct of the poses that follow, stretching is not the goal, so resist any temptation to coax your body into a deeper stretch here. This reminds me of the words of Judith Hanson Lasater, who I studied restorative yoga with, when she says that restorative yoga is not about stretching, it's about opening. Allow your body to ease into each pose and be supported by your props. Use this sequence to encourage the relaxation response and enhance your recovery.

Legs up the wall with optional wall wide angle pose and bound angle pose variations

---

DURATION: 2 to 10 minutes
SUGGESTED PROPS: A wall, two to three pillows, two to three cushions, one to three blankets, one soft scarf or eye mask (optional: a belt)

See pp. 66–71 for full instructions.

Legs up the wall – wide angle variation
From Legs up the wall, take your legs apart as far as your hips will comfortably allow.

Legs up the wall – bound angle variation
From Legs up the wall, bring the soles of your feet together, creating a diamond shape with your legs, and slide the outside edges of your feet down the wall towards your hips (as far down the wall as feels comfortable).

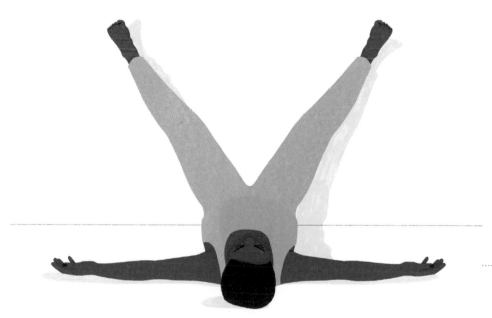

Sequence for post-workout

SUGGESTED PROPS: Access to a wall, two to three pillows, two to three cushions, one or two blankets, one soft scarf or eye mask (optional: a belt)

1 **Supported half-frog pose** (2 to 5 minutes on each side – up to 10 minutes in total)
   See pp. 59–60 for full instructions.
2 **Supported bridge pose** (2 to 5 minutes)
   See pp. 64–5 for full instructions.
3 **Supported reclining twist – version A or B** (2 to 5 minutes on each side)
   Remember to allow your abdomen to be soft. You might notice your navel gently rising and falling.
   See pp. 49–52 for full instructions.
4 **Legs up the wall, as above with optional wide angle variation and/or bound angle variation** (2 to 10 minutes)
   See pp. 66–71 for full instructions.

Post-practice reflection: I am grateful for the body that I have because …

Rest + Calm

Rest session for **computer** or **smartphone posture**

Computer and smartphone posture – something that more and more of us are impacted by. Even if you don't use a computer or smartphone on a regular basis, the chances are that if you're sitting a lot you probably find yourself in rounded back, head forward position more often than you would like, resulting in discomfort and muscle tightness. The following is a one-blanket restorative practice to help create a more open feeling in the upper body. You will just need one blanket rolled into a long sausage shape. Alternatively, you could use a bath towel.

If you don't have time to practise all three of the poses here, feel free to pick the one that you feel will be of most benefit and do that.

Supported fish pose – version A – on a blanket roll (2 to 5 minutes)
Place your blanket roll lengthways on the floor – the roll should ideally be long enough to reach from the base of your spine to the top of your head. Sit on the floor with one end of the blanket roll behind you. Bring the soles of your feet to the floor and place your palms down on the floor by your hips. Carefully lie back on the blanket roll so that it rests along your spine and the back of your head is supported. Rest your arms by your sides with your palms facing up. For more opening, move your arms further away from your torso or rest your arms in cactus shape.

With the soles of your feet still on the floor, allow your legs and feet to be approximately hip-width apart. Alternatively, take your feet wider than hip-width apart and bring your knees towards each other.

When you are ready to exit this pose, carefully roll off your blanket on to one side. Rest here for a few breaths before guiding yourself up to sitting.

Supported fish pose – version B – on a blanket roll (2 to 5 minutes)
Place your blanket roll horizontally on the ground. Sit on the floor with a long side of the blanket roll behind you. Bring the soles of your feet to the floor and place your palms down on the floor by your hips. Carefully lie back on the blanket roll until it rests just below your armpits. Allow the back of your head to rest on the floor. Take your arms out wide (approximately

shoulder height) with palms facing up. Alternatively, rest your arms in a cactus shape.

With the soles of your feet still on the floor, allow your legs and feet to be approximately hip-width apart. Alternatively, take your feet wider and bring your knees towards each other.

When you're ready to exit this pose, carefully roll completely off your blanket on to one side. Rest here for a few breaths before guiding yourself up to sitting.

Supported bridge – on a blanket roll (2 to 5 minutes)
Place your blanket roll horizontally on the ground. Sit on a long side of the blanket roll. Bring the soles of your feet to the floor and place your palms down on the floor behind you. Let your arms support you as you press your palms and the soles of your feet on to the floor, lifting your hips. Slide your hips slightly forward and rest your sacrum (the bony back of your pelvis, below your lower back curve) on to the blanket roll. Use your arms to lower your back on to the floor into your Supported bridge position. Take your arms out wide (approximately shoulder height) with palms facing up or rest your arms in a cactus shape.

With the soles of your feet still on the floor, allow your legs and feet to be approximately hip-width apart.

When you're ready to exit this pose, press the soles of your feet on to the floor to lift your hips. Slide your blanket roll away from your body and lower your sacrum on to the floor. Allow your knees to move right and left (*Windscreen wipers – see* pp. 27–8). Then roll over to one side and rest there for a few breaths until you feel ready to come to a sitting position.

Post-practice reflection: The head down, rounded back nature of 'computer posture' can leave the body feeling quite 'closed'. How does your body feel now after this practice? And where in your life can you invite more openness?

part 2

calm

How to find calm

In this section you will find a range of suggestions for away from the yoga mat to help you find calm in your day. Some are grounded in yoga, while others are general practical tips, including some research-backed ideas.

The power of breath

Breathing is the first thing we do when we enter the world, and the last thing we do as we leave. An average resting adult takes about 23,000 breaths per day and for as long as each of us is here, our breath is the one constant we have. Yet many of us do not breathe effectively. Without realising it, perhaps due to physical or emotional tension, how we hold our bodies or unconscious habit, our breathing is shallow. But it wasn't always that way. Watching babies breathe is a reminder that we too began knowing how to breathe well.

As more and more people come to understand the benefits of breathing well, it is of no surprise that breathwork has been increasingly gaining in popularity over the past few years. But did you know that many of these breathing practices originate from yoga? Specifically, pranayama, the fourth of the eight limbs of yoga (*see* p. 19).

What is pranayama?

The most common translation from Sanskrit of 'prana' is 'life force', so pranayama is most often described as the practice of breath – life force or energy – control. This is because 'yama' on its own means 'control' or 'restraint'. However, 'ayama' is the opposite (expansion), so, pranayama can be described as the practice of life force (breath) expansion. In yoga tradition, breath is seen as the vehicle that carries our life force or life energy, so, by consciously working with our breath we support the flow of prana – life force – through our bodies.

Your breath as an anchor

One of the benefits of breathing practices is that you can usually do them anywhere at any time to help ground and calm yourself and often no one else need know what you're doing. Some of the breathing practices that follow can be easily incorporated into your restorative yoga practice, but for those times when you're not able to do a restorative yoga practice, and for anyone who has absolutely no intention of doing a yoga posture ever, the breath on its own is powerful and effective.

Deep breathing stimulates the vagus nerve, soothing physical and emotional stress, and calming both body and mind. Related to this, numerous studies have demonstrated the benefits of breathing practices for anxiety, depression, PTSD, asthma and more. For example, the findings of a 2019 study showed that pranayama improved sleep quality in people with obstructive sleep apnoea and research from King's College London found that deep breathing, particularly at a rate of six breaths per minute, can help people with pain management.

In the REST section of this book we touched on some breathing practices, in particular 1:1 breathing (sama vritti), where the inhalation is the same length as the exhalation. This is one example of how, just as you can energise yourself by consciously adjusting your breathing, you can calm yourself too.

Although there are many breathing practices you can do, the ones that follow are among some of the most accessible, calming techniques. There are some practices that involve breath retention (holding the breath), but for some people this may bring on feelings of anxiety. If this is your experience, then please avoid doing it. If in doubt, 1:1 breathing is a good place to start. Then you can explore some of the others from there. As always, practise with ahimsa – without force or strain – and treat yourself with kindness. At the end of your breathing practice, do take a few moments to observe any effect it has had.

1:1 breathing

For 1:1 breathing or sama vritti, aim to inhale for a count of four and exhale for a count of four. If this feels too much for your breath capacity, then start lower, so inhale for a count of two and exhale for a count of two.

1:2 breathing

For 1:2 breathing, aim to move towards your exhale being twice as long as your exhale. For example, if your inhale lasts for a count of four, allow your exhale to last for a count of eight. If this feels too much for your breath capacity, then start lower, so inhale for a count of two and exhale for a count of four. If this still feels challenging, start with 1:1 breathing and play with allowing your exhale to be slightly longer than your inhale, so inhale for a count of two and exhale for a count of three. Extending the exhale can be helpful for balancing anxiety.

Diaphragmatic breathing

This is best practised lying down, particularly if you're new to diaphragmatic breathing as it makes it easier to physically feel the rise and fall of your breath. If you are lying on your back you may find it helpful to place one hand on your chest and your other hand on your belly. As you inhale slowly through your nose, you may notice your hands rise. As you exhale you may notice your hands fall. As you continue to slowly inhale and exhale through your nose, you may notice your chest become a little more still as your belly gently moves up and down. As you inhale, your belly gently rises as your diaphragm moves downward and air comes into your lungs. As you exhale, your belly gently falls as your diaphragm relaxes and air moves out of your lungs. Continue this for several rounds.

You can also do this lying on your front (*see Face-down relaxation pose on pp. 57–8*), where you can feel the contact and rise and fall of your front-body on the ground as you inhale and exhale.

A NOTE ON DIAPHRAGMATIC BREATHING

Although the belly may rise and fall as a result of the movement of the diaphragm itself, the aim is not to force the belly to expand. When you're newer to this practice it is usually easier to gauge via the movement of the belly and it is an effective way to promote calm, as well as massaging the abdominal organs. However, with practice and over time, as your diaphragm moves and your lungs fill with more air on the inhalation (the opposite of shallow upper chest breathing), you will become more aware of your ribcage spreading in all directions and your belly will move less.

Alternate nostril breathing

Nadi shodhana pranayama, as alternate nostril breathing is also known, is a balancing practice. Nadi means 'channel' or 'flow of energy' while shodhana means 'purification'. The two main subtle energy channels (nadis) involved here are ida, associated with the right side of the brain and left side of the body, and pingala, associated with the left side of the brain and the right side of the body. While ida is known for cooling and calming, pingala is known for heating and activating.

With regard to breathing, if the breath is stronger through the right nostril, pingala is more active. If the breath is stronger through the left nostril then ida is more active. It is normal for one nostril to be more active or dominant than the other and this usually changes throughout the day.

The goal of this practice is to help balance our energy flow and research has shown that it lowers stress, heart rate and can have a positive effect on cardiovascular function.

Psychic alternate nostril breathing

Alternate nostril breathing can be and is usually practised with a hand mudra, where the thumb and fourth finger are used to open and close the nostrils (for more detail on *mudras see* pp. 142–5). I have shared some practice guidance on this below. However, I am very keen to share this version – psychic alternate nostril breathing – with you too as not only is it easier to practise while you are in a restorative yoga pose such as Supported reclining bound angle, it also is a way of practising alternate nostril breathing anywhere without announcing it to the world (for instance, when you're sitting on a bus or train). I've practised this many a time on delayed journeys to calm agitation. Also, another practical reason that you might want to opt for this version is if you suffer with allergies or have nasal obstructions that make closing the nostrils unadvisable or uncomfortable.

Start by becoming aware of the flow of air moving in and out through both nostrils. Do this for five breaths.

Guide your awareness to your left nostril and visualise the breath moving in through just the left nostril as you inhale and the breath moving out through the right nostril as you exhale. On your next inhale visualise the breath moving in through just the right nostril and then out through the left nostril as you exhale – this is one round of psychic alternate nostril breathing. Continue – on your inhale visualise the breath moving in through the left nostril and as you exhale visualise the breath moving out through the right. Continue with this breathing pattern for several rounds of breath, ending by exhaling through your left nostril.

Practising alternate nostril breathing with a mudra

Usually this is practised with breath retention (holding the breath at certain intervals), but I would suggest that if you are new to this begin by focusing on just the inhales and exhales through each nostril instead. The instructions below are without breath retention. (You may wish to avoid this practice if you have a cold, flu or nasal obstructions.)

Start by sitting or kneeling comfortably with a tall spine. With eyes closed or your gaze softened to one spot, breathe in and out normally through the nose several times.

Place one hand underneath your nostrils and breathe on to your hand to see which nostril feels more active.

Rest your left hand comfortably on your left thigh (or take *chin mudra* or *jnana mudra* – see pp. 143–4). Bring your right hand into one of the following mudras.

Nasagra mudra: Rest the tips of your index and middle fingers gently on your eyebrow centre and hover your right thumb over your right nostril and right ring finger over your left nostril.

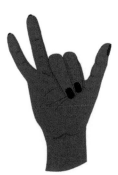

Vishnu mudra: Bend your right index and middle finger, bring the tips of those fingers to the centre of your right palm and hover your right thumb over your right nostril and right ring finger over your left nostril.

For whichever mudra you choose, you will be using your right thumb and right ring finger to open and close your nostrils. Your right little finger can be relaxed throughout.

Depending on which nostril was more active, softly close the opposite nostril and breathe in and out through the more active nostril five times. After five breaths, release the nostril that was closed, pause and take a breath or two through both nostrils before repeating five single nostril breaths through the opposite nostril.

If you weren't able to tell which nostril was more active, then gently close the right nostril with your right thumb and breathe in and out through the left nostril five times. After five breaths, release the right nostril and take a breath or two through both nostrils. Then softly close the left nostril with your right ring finger and breathe in and out through your right nostril five times. After five single nostril breaths, release the right nostril and breathe in and out through both nostrils five times.

Now adopt your mudra again. Softly close your right nostril with your right thumb and inhale slowly and steadily through your left nostril. Softly close your left nostril (with your right ring finger) and release your right nostril. Exhale slowly and steadily through your right nostril. Let your inhales and exhales be equal in length. Inhale through your right nostril. Softly close your right nostril (with your right thumb) and release closure of your left. Exhale through your left nostril.

This completes one round.

Repeat this for five to 10 rounds, focusing on your steady inhales and exhales. End by exhaling through your left nostril. When you're finished, rest both arms and breathe in and out normally through the nostrils for several breaths.

Whether you are practising alternate nostril breathing with your hand mudra or psychic alternate nostril breathing, aim for five minutes of focused breathing. When you feel comfortable with five minutes then you can choose to extend your practice, gradually working up to 15 minutes.

Left nostril breathing

If your mind is feeling restless, try left nostril breathing or chandra bhedana pranayama. Translated as 'Piercing the moon', this practice can also be helpful in the evening when you want to wind down.

As with alternate nostril breathing, you will use your right thumb and ring finger to help control the flow of air through the nostrils. The difference is that you will inhale only through the left nostril and exhale only through the right nostril. Also, as you learned with alternate nostril breathing, the left nostril is linked with ida nadi. As the 'cooling' side, the left nostril is also related to the moon (chandra), whereas the right 'heating' side is related to the sun (surya). (As with alternate nostril breathing, you may wish to avoid this practice if you have a cold, flu or nasal obstructions.)

Breathe steadily in and out through both nostrils a few times.

With your right hand in nasagra mudra or vishnu mudra, softly close your right nostril with your right thumb and inhale through your left nostril. Softly close your left nostril with your right ring finger, release the right nostril and exhale through your right nostril.

Continue this same breathing pattern – inhaling through your left nostril and exhaling through your right nostril – for several rounds of breath, aiming for one to three minutes. When you feel comfortable with this, you can choose to extend your practice up to five minutes.

Bee breath

Research on bhramari pranayama or bee breath – known as this because the sound of the exhale is similar to that of a humming bee – has shown that five minutes of this breathing practice can encourage parasympathetic dominance on the cardiovascular system by helping to reduce blood pressure and heart rate. The humming sound of the breath can also be helpful for dampening mental chatter, so this breathing practice is one to opt for if your mind is very busy. You may also want to do this practice when you are getting ready for sleep.

Like alternate nostril breathing, bee breath can be practised with or without a mudra.

Bee breath without a mudra

With your eyes closed or your gaze softened to one spot, breathe in and out several times.

Take a deep, steady inhale. As you exhale steadily, make a humming sound (as though trying to say 'mmmm') with your facial muscles and jaw relaxed, and your mouth closed. Allow your humming sound to be relaxed (so that you are not forcing the sound or the volume) and to last for the full duration of your exhale.

Repeat this for five breaths.

During each exhale, notice how the vibration of your humming sounds feels, particularly in your face and head. When you have completed five breaths take a few steady regular breaths before gently opening your eyes (if they were closed).

Once you feel comfortable with five breaths, you may wish to extend the duration of your practice, eventually working up to five minutes.

If you're using this practice as part of your preparation for sleep, allow your humming sound to be low-pitched and not too loud.

Bee breath with shanmukhi mudra

This version of bee breath uses shanmukhi mudra which represents 'closing the six gates of perception' and involves covering the eyes and blocking the ears ('shan' means 'six' and 'mukhi' means 'face'). If you experience claustrophobia, anxiety or depression then avoid this version.

Sitting or kneeling with a tall spine, breathe in and out several times. Spread your fingers to come into shanmukhi mudra:

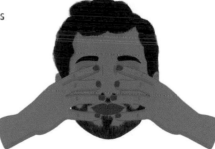

- Place the tips of your little fingers below your bottom lip
- Place the tips of your ring fingers above your top lip just below your nose
- Place the tips of your middle fingers on each side of your nose
- Place the tips of each index finger on your eyelids to close each eye
- Place the tips of your thumbs over each ear, blocking out sound

Allow the pressure from your fingers on your face and ears to be gentle and your elbows to move back.

Take a deep, steady inhale. As you exhale steadily, make a humming sound (as though trying to say 'mmmm'). As with the mudra-free version, allow your humming sound to be relaxed (so that you are not forcing the sound or the volume) and to last for the full duration of your exhale.

Repeat this for five breaths.

During each exhale, notice how the vibration of your humming sounds feels, particularly in your face and head.

When you have completed your five breaths, release the mudra and take a few regular breaths before gently opening your eyes.

Once you feel comfortable with five breaths, you may wish to extend the duration of your practice, eventually working up to five minutes.

Silent bee breath

This version is for when you would like to practise bee breath but are in an environment or situation where you are unable to or do not want to make the humming sound. This is much the same as bee breath without a mudra, but silent.

If you are safely able to close your eyes and would like to, please do so. Otherwise, soften your gaze to somewhere in your eyeline.

Take a deep, steady inhale. As you exhale steadily, imagine that you are making a relaxed humming sound (as though internally saying 'mmmm' to yourself). Allow your internal humming to last for the full duration of your exhale.

During each exhale, observe any sensations that may be arising, particularly in your face and head.

Repeat this for five breaths.

Once you feel comfortable with five breaths, you may wish to extend the duration of your practice, eventually working up to five minutes.

Three-part exhale

Also known as viloma pranayama – 'vi' means 'against' and 'loma' means 'hair', so viloma is commonly translated as 'against the wave' or 'against the natural flow' – there are three versions of the three-part exhale: interrupted inhale, interrupted exhale and interrupted inhalation and exhalation. The second version, interrupted exhale, is said to be anxiety-soothing and calming for the mind, so it's this version of viloma we will particularly focus on.

Allow your breathing, as well as your facial muscles, jaw and neck, to be as relaxed as possible throughout.

Breathe in and out through the nose steadily several times.

Take a deep inhale, filling the lungs.

Exhale a third of the breath, then pause.

Exhale another third of the breath, then pause.

Exhale the final third of the breath, then pause.

Expel any remaining air from your lungs. Once your lungs feel completely empty, pause before taking another deep inhale, to repeat your three-part exhale. Aim for five rounds.

When you feel comfortable with five rounds, you may wish to extend the duration of your practice, eventually working up to 10 rounds.

Once your practice is complete, take several regular, steady breaths and observe how you feel.

Ocean breathing

Ujjayi pranayama is commonly translated as 'victorious breath', but this practice is also known as ocean breathing because of the gentle sound of ocean waves it creates.

It is one of the most common breathing practices used alongside more active yoga posture styles and is a warming breath, so this is worth bearing in mind if you don't wish to create additional heat in your body.

Begin by taking a few regular, steady breaths in and out of the nose.

Take a deep inhale through the nose. As you exhale through your mouth, make a gentle 'haa' sound. It may be helpful to imagine that you are trying to fog up a mirror in front of you with your breath. Repeat this several times.

On your next breath, repeat the above steps, but this time, exhale with your mouth closed so that there is a soft, whispering sound to your breath. Allow your throat to stay as relaxed as possible throughout – just a slight constriction at the back of the throat is enough. Let your inhale and exhale be approximately the same length.

Continue with your ocean breathing for two minutes. When you feel comfortable with this you may wish to extend the duration of your practice up to five minutes.

One-minute re-set: triangle breath

In this practice, which is useful if you feel particularly short on time, you will be following this breathing pattern:

- Inhale for four
- Hold for four
- Exhale for seven

Start by visualising a triangle. You can close your eyes if that makes it easier. As an option, you may wish to see each side of the triangle as a different colour as you breathe.

Begin at the bottom left corner of the triangle.

Inhale for four counts as you trace the first side of the triangle.

Gently hold your breath for four counts as you trace the second side of the triangle.

Exhale for seven counts as you trace the third side of the triangle.

For a short practice repeat this breathing sequence, visualising your triangle four times. If you would like to extend your practice, continue to repeat this sequence for up to five minutes.

Box breathing

In this practice you will be following this breathing pattern:

- Inhale for four
- Hold for four
- Exhale for four
- Hold for four

Start by visualising a square. You can close your eyes if that makes it easier. As an option, you might wish to see each side of the box as a different colour as you breathe.

Begin at the bottom left corner of the box.

Inhale for four counts as you trace up the left side of the square.

Hold your breath for four counts as you trace the top side of the square.

Exhale for four counts as you trace down the right side of the square.

Gently hold your breath for four counts as you trace the bottom side of the square.

For a short practice repeat this breathing sequence, visualising your square four times. If you would like to extend your practice, continue to repeat this sequence for up to five minutes.

4-7-8 breathing

This breathing practice is similar to box breathing and was developed by Dr Andrew Weil MD, in part via his experience of pranayama. Dr Weil claims that over his decades of experience 4-7-8 breathing has shown itself to be an incredibly effective way to manage stress and anxiety. This can be useful as part of your sleep preparation too and it's also said to be helpful for getting back to sleep if you wake up in the night.

In this practice you will be following this breathing pattern:

- Inhale for four.
- Hold for seven.
- Exhale for eight.

Begin by taking several regular breaths in and out of the nose. Inhale through your nose for four counts. Gently hold your breath for seven counts. Exhale through your mouth audibly for eight counts. Repeat this breathing pattern four times, twice a day.

If you are practising 4-7-8 breathing daily, Dr Weil suggests sticking with four repetitions, twice a day for the first month. After a month, you can choose to extend your practice by eventually working up to a maximum of eight repetitions per practice.

Grounding techniques to promote calm

Here are some suggestions for helping to restore your equilibrium.
I encourage you to experiment with each of them if you can, to discover
whether you have a favourite. You might also find that you like to adopt
different techniques for different situations.

Give yourself a hug

While you may be familiar with the feel-good effects of a hug from a loved
one or friend, did you know that wrapping your arms around yourself can
be good for you too? For all sorts of reasons it is not always possible to hug
those who are dear to us. More recently, the pandemic has kept so many of
us apart, whether by a distance of a couple of metres or thousands of miles.
In fact, since Covid-19 more of us have experienced touch starvation, so it
can be reassuring and helpful to know that you can harness the power of
a hug in your own hands (and arms!).

TOUCH STARVATION

The absence of touch from other living beings is known as touch
starvation. Since the Covid-19 pandemic and the implementation
of social distancing, casual, friendly touch such as handshakes or
hugs are either few and far between or non-existent for many of
us. Touch is important for mental and physical health – research
from 2014 found that the absence of regular human touch can be
detrimental. Even if you are someone who does not like to be
touched by other people, you may still experience the effects of
touch starvation, which can manifest as stress, loneliness, feelings
of isolation, depression, anxiety and poor sleep. Self-touch, such
as giving yourself a hug, is one way to address this (see pp. 139–140
for more suggestions).

According to research, just a few of the benefits of hugging yourself are:

* Reduction of cortisol (stress hormone)
* Increase in the production of oxytocin (love hormone)
* Reduction in pain
* Improved mood
* More compassion towards yourself

HOW TO GET THERE: Fold your arms across the front of your chest. Allow each hand to rest on your shoulders or on your upper arms.

Alternatively, you might prefer to fold your arms around your abdomen and allow your fingers to curl around the sides of your tummy or waist. See what feels like the most comfortable, soothing option for you.

Hold your hug for as long as it feels good.

While you are there, think about the type of hug you want and need in that moment. For instance, you might want to squeeze your shoulders or the sides of your body to make your hug tighter. Or you might wish to gently stroke the backs of your shoulders or arms. If hugging around the chest, you might like to nestle your head into your arms. You might even like to gently sway back and forth in your hug. There is no one right way. The right way in this instance is what feels best for you.

Soothing away touch starvation

As well as giving yourself a hug, here are some other suggestions for addressing touch starvation.

Weighting: As mentioned in the *REST* section and featured in some of the restorative practices, placing weight on the body may be calming and grounding if you're experiencing anxiety and soothing if you're experiencing depression. If you have ever used weighted blankets, this idea may be familiar to you. If you do have a weighted blanket, you can place it on your body or wrap it around you. Even cocooning yourself in a regular blanket can be soothing, as can placing folded blankets or similar on your body. All the better if you have time to do this while lying down in a restorative yoga pose (see the *Rest session for anxiety* and the *Rest session for depression* in the *REST* section for starting points).

Tissue work: Rolling a tennis ball over the sole of your feet (and also rubbing your feet) can help to stimulate the vagus nerve. You can also lie back on a tennis ball, placing it under an area that feels tight, such as just above the shoulder blade near the top of the back. This can also be done against a wall instead of lying down, although the sensation of the ball itself can be quite intense, so you may want to place something soft, like a towel or blanket, over the ball.

Self-massage: Giving yourself a gentle neck massage or hand massage can be soothing. Related to this, an alternative could be mindfully applying moisturiser to your skin after a shower or bath.

ASMR: Autonomous sensory meridian response (ASMR) relates to the experience of tingling sensations – usually starting with pleasant sensations in the crown of the head before moving down the body – resulting from gentle touch, such as having your hair washed, or listening to particular sounds, such as whispering or rainfall. While for some people these kinds of sounds might be annoying, for others they are incredibly relaxing and calming. It is likely that you will already know which group you are part of. Research findings indicate that ASMR may have therapeutic benefits for mental and physical health and it is believed that these sounds stimulate the part of the brain that processes touch, so you may wish to consider seeking out ASMR videos or recordings online.

Five-four-three-two-one

This is a simple, effective grounding technique that can be helpful if you are experiencing anxiety, a racing mind or feeling overwhelmed by emotions. With the five-four-three-two-one method you use your senses to guide your awareness to the present moment.

HOW TO GET THERE: Start by noticing your breathing. Begin to deepen your breath and allow your inhale and exhale to be steady (1:1 or 1:2 breathing).

See – notice five things that you can see. Look around your environment. Slowly take in what you see. For example, this could be really observing the shape of your fingers, the outline of the leaves on a houseplant or the form of an item of furniture. If you're outside or by a window you might acknowledge the sky or the characteristics of a particular tree or building.

Touch – notice four things you can touch. What is there in your environment that you can touch? It could be parts of your body. It could be the ground beneath your feet or the texture of an item of clothing you are wearing. If you're sitting at a desk, it could be a pen, a computer, phone or the desk itself. If you're outside in a green space, it could be a tree or plant. The items you touch could be large or small.

Hear – notice three things you can hear. Guide your awareness to sounds outside your body, so rather than focusing on, say, the sound of your breathing or your tummy rumbling, acknowledge the sounds around you instead. This could be a clock ticking, traffic or birds singing.

Smell – notice two things you can smell. Depending on where you are, this one might be more of a challenge. You could start by focusing on the smell of your own skin and any smell in the air. This could also be a particular scent you like that is within your reach, such as your favourite perfume, aftershave or essential oil.

Taste – notice one thing you can taste. This could be the lingering taste on your tongue of the last thing you ate, but if you're unable to taste anything in that moment, then you could think of your favourite thing to taste. Alternatively, rather than noticing one thing you can taste, you could acknowledge one positive thing about yourself.

End with a few conscious, deep breaths and give yourself credit for doing this – acknowledge that you were able to successfully complete this practice.

Try this exercise a few times when you're in a calm state to familiarise yourself with the process. That way, when you turn to it in an anxious or overwhelmed state you will know what to do.

Keeping your eyes open throughout may help you feel more at ease. If you're on your own and feel comfortable to speak aloud, you might also like to state each item you're taking in and notice how it feels to do this.

You may find that going through this five-four-three-two-one process once is enough to leave you feeling more grounded and present, but please feel free to repeat it as many times as needed. With regular practice of this technique, you may notice that you become less likely to be swept along by worst-case-scenario thinking and feel more in control.

Earthing

When was the last time you walked or stood barefoot on the grass? Living in a busy city with no garden and temperamental weather means this is not something I get to do very often, but when the weather is good, or I am visiting sunnier climes, I really make the most of the opportunities to feel my feet on the earth.

Earthing (also known as grounding) involves the skin being in contact with natural ground (so your carpet at home doesn't count). That means you can also experience earthing by lying down on grass or walking or lying down on sand.

Though scientific studies on earthing are currently limited, research from 2018 showed that grounding may have a positive effect on pain and quality of life overall and according to the findings of a small study from 2015, an hour of grounding therapy can improve mood.

If you are fortunate enough to have access to a garden at your home, then this is something you can take full advantage of. Otherwise, when you are next able to get out to a safe green space or a beach give earthing a try.

Mudras for calm

According to yoga philosophy, there are 72,000 nadis (subtle energy pathways) throughout our bodies. Many of these energy pathways end in our hands, so by holding our hands in specific positions – or gestures – coupled with focused awareness we create an energy seal – a mudra – between nadis.

The human body could be described as a universe within itself and so the five elements of the universe exist within each of us too. In Ayurveda ('the science of life', often referred to as yoga's sister science) it is believed that the human body is comprised of these five elements. Each finger and thumb relates to a particular element:

- Thumb – fire (agni)
- Index finger – air (vayu)
- Middle finger – ether/space (akasha)
- Ring finger – earth (prithvi)
- Little finger – water (jala)

With this in mind, hand mudras (hasta mudras) can help to balance the energies of the elements and there are many hand mudras you can practise for different purposes. Here are just a few mudras that can be helpful for promoting calm. It is normal to not 'feel' much at first, especially if mudras are totally new to you, but choosing which of the following most resonates with you and being willing to practise is a great place to start. Stay in each mudra for as long as feels comfortable unless otherwise stated. Remember to allow your breath to be smooth and steady.

If in doubt, stay with your 1:1 breathing.

Chin mudra – gesture of consciousness

This is one of the mudras most people will probably recognise from images of yoga practitioners meditating. This mudra promotes calmness and peace, and it involves joining the thumb's fire element with the index finger's air element.

Find a comfortable sitting position. With your palms facing up, rest the backs of your hands on your knees or thighs. Create a circle by touching the tip of your thumb to the tip of your index finger. Alternatively, you can bring the tip of your index finger to the base of the thumb, forming a smaller circle. Allow your other fingers to be straight, yet slightly apart and relaxed.

Aim to hold this mudra for five minutes, although it's OK to start with a shorter duration and work your way up to five minutes. When you feel comfortable with five minutes, you can choose to extend your practice to up to 15 minutes.

Jnana mudra – gesture of wisdom

This is similar to chin mudra, but is practised with the palms facing down, which promotes grounding. Follow the same steps as chin mudra, but with your palms resting down your legs.

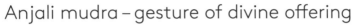

Aim to hold this mudra for five minutes, although it's OK to start with a shorter duration and work your way up to five minutes. When you feel comfortable with five minutes, you can choose to extend your practice to up to 15 minutes.

Anjali mudra – gesture of divine offering

This is another of the most recognisable mudras. Anjali mudra promotes a calm mind and improved focus as well as relief from stress.

Begin with your palms open, facing up, as though you are making an offering with your hands. Slowly bring your palms together into a prayer position and move your hands to the centre of your chest with your fingers pointing upwards. Repeat this movement of opening and closing your palms a few times. When you feel ready, settle into your anjali mudra (palms together in a prayer position) with your hands at the centre of your chest.

Sukham mudra – gesture of stress relief

The clue is in the name of this mudra. This is ideal to do at the start of your day, particularly if your schedule feels overwhelming.

Find a comfortable sitting position. With your palms facing up, touch the tip of your right thumb to the ends of your little and middle fingers. With your left hand, press your thumb on to the nail of your little finger. Allow the other fingers on each hand to be straight, yet relaxed.

Aim to hold this mudra for two minutes.

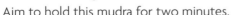

Ganesha mudra – gesture of remover of obstacles

Ganesha is the Hindu deity who is known as the remover of obstacles. Ease from tension and stress are just two of the benefits of this mudra.

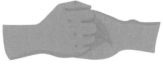

Place your right palm in front of your chest with your right fingertips pointing to the left. Place your left palm on your right palm with your left fingertips pointing to the right. Clasp your hands by hooking your fingers and thumbs together. You can keep your hands at chest height (with elbows out) or rest your hands in your lap.

Shakti mudra – gesture of divine power

If you've been experiencing stress-induced insomnia, then this mudra may be of help. Translated from Sanskrit, 'shakti' means 'power'. Shakti is also another name for Hindu deity Durga, the goddess of strength and power.

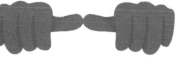

Find a comfortable sitting position. Bring your thumbs into each palm then wrap your index and middle fingers over each thumb. Bring the tip of each ring finger together and the tip of each little finger together.

Once you feel comfortable with shakti mudra, this can be practised for up to 15 minutes.

Agni shakti mudra – gesture of fire energy

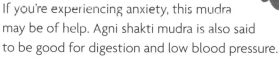

If you're experiencing anxiety, this mudra may be of help. Agni shakti mudra is also said to be good for digestion and low blood pressure.

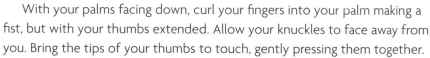

With your palms facing down, curl your fingers into your palm making a fist, but with your thumbs extended. Allow your knuckles to face away from you. Bring the tips of your thumbs to touch, gently pressing them together.

The benefits of body scanning

A body scan is a type of meditation. Aside from bringing you into the present moment, body scanning is a particularly helpful way of checking in with yourself. Research has shown that body scanning can be helpful for adults experiencing chronic pain as well as easing anxiety and stress.

There are various kinds of body scan you can do – there is no one right way to do it – and here are two examples for you to try. The first is a shorter, basic systematic relaxation body scan, which is ideal for when you have less time or are, say, sitting at your desk. The second is a longer practice that involves bringing a little more awareness to each part of the body. This is for when you have more time and you might even wish to use this as part of your sleep preparation. As you become more accustomed to the practice, you will be able to guide yourself with ease, making body scanning accessible to you whenever you need it.

For each of the practices below, allow yourself to be in a comfortable position, either seated or lying down. As an option, you may wish to incorporate the *Tense and release* exercise from the *REST* section beforehand (*see* pp. 30–1). When you're ready to close your practice, allow yourself to take your time as you gradually reorient to your surroundings. If your mind wanders during your practice, that's OK and normal – guide your awareness back to your body and continue where you left off, without any judgement. As ever, this is not about perfection – that's why we call it 'practice'.

Body scan systematic relaxation

Find your steady, comfortable breathing rhythm and begin to observe the rise and fall of your breath. With each exhale, feel the tension in your physical body softening a little more. With each exhale, release any tension in your jaw, the spaces behind your jaw, the muscles around your ears, your scalp, your temples, your forehead, eye muscles, cheeks, neck and throat, shoulders, upper arms, lower arms, hands, all your fingers, your upper torso, your lower torso, your abdomen, hips, thighs, lower legs, feet, all of your toes, the whole body right and left, the whole body front and back, the whole body, the whole body together, the whole body at ease.

Allow yourself to be here for as long as you wish – simply rest and breathe.

Body scan meditation

Allow your breath to be as steady and comfortable as possible, with the weight of your body completely supported by the surface you're resting on, and begin to become aware of the parts of your body that are in contact with that surface. Maybe you notice the texture of the surface where your physical body is resting.

Now gently guide your awareness to the rise and fall of your breathing. Don't control your breath, just watch and sense the body breathing. Observe the quality of your breath. Is it full and deep? Is it shallow? There might be an awareness of parts of the body moving with your breath. For instance, maybe there's an awareness of the abdomen gently rising and falling, or the side ribs gently expanding and contracting.

On your next breath, as you inhale, visualise the breath moving from the tips of your toes to the crown of your head. As you exhale, visualise the breath moving from the crown of your head to the tips of your toes. Continue with this visualisation for a few breaths – inhaling breath from the tips of the toes to the crown of the head and exhaling breath from the crown of the head to the tips of the toes.

On your next exhale, allow your awareness to gently rest on your feet. Soon you will begin to guide the focus of your attention to different parts of your body to observe if there are any sensations that arise in those parts of the body. The sensations may be on the surface of the body or inside the body. If there is no sensation, then note that. Neither is right or wrong. As your awareness travels around the body, allow yourself to pause at each part of the body as you observe. Allow your breath to remain steady.

Notice any sensations in your toes, the soles of both feet, the heels, the tops of the feet, the ankles. On your next exhale, guide the focus of your attention to the calves, noticing any sensation in the calves and then the shins. As you exhale fully, guide your attention to the knees, observing any sensation at the knees. As you exhale, guide your attention to the thighs. What do you notice? Exhale fully and guide your awareness to the pelvis. Notice any sensations at the right hip, the left hip and in the whole pelvic bowl. Maybe there's an awareness of the organs here. Exhale fully and guide your awareness to the lower back, the mid back, the upper back and the whole spine, right shoulder and shoulder blade, left shoulder and shoulder blade, observing any sensations arising in the back and shoulders. Exhale fully and guide your awareness to the abdomen, noticing any sensations arising here. Exhale fully and guide your awareness to the chest, observing.

Exhale fully and guide your awareness to your hands – the back of your hands, the palms and all the fingers, noticing any sensations. Exhale fully and guide your attention to the wrists and lower arms, observing the elbows and upper arms, noticing sensations in the elbows and upper arms. Exhale fully and guide your awareness to the neck, observing any sensations in the neck. Exhale fully and guide your awareness to the whole face and head, noticing any sensations in the chin, jaw, lower lip, upper lip, nose, right cheek, left cheek, right ear, left ear, right eye, left eye, right eyebrow, left eyebrow, space between the eyebrows, forehead, right temple, left temple, scalp and the back of the head, observing any sensations in the whole face and head.

On your next exhale, visualise the breath moving from the crown of your head to the tips of your toes. As you inhale, visualise the breath moving from the tips of the toes to the crown of the head. Exhale as you visualise the breath moving from the crown of the head to the tips of the toes. As you continue with this visualisation for several breaths, observe whether there is any difference to the quality of your breath or how you feel compared to at the beginning of this practice. Then let go of this visualisation and allow the breath and body to just be. Allow yourself to be here for as long as you wish. Simply rest and breathe.

Yoga nidra

Yoga nidra has a special place in my heart. I feel this is because there are ways in which restorative yoga and yoga nidra overlap. Both practices:

- promote deep rest and rejuvenation
- can guide you to a pratyahara state ('withdrawal of the senses')
- have the capacity to create the conditions for more clarity, awakening and coming back home to yourself
- do not require previous experience of yoga

But what is yoga nidra?

Yoga nidra is commonly known as 'yogic sleep'. First and foremost, it is a state. The state of yoga nidra relates to pratyahara, the fifth of the eight limbs of yoga (see p. 19), but it is also described as a technique. However, it was not until during a training with teacher Tracee Stanley that I learned Yoga Nidra is also a goddess.

The technique is a form of guided meditation that is deeply restful, which can (although it is not always guaranteed to) lead the practitioner to a state of yoga nidra, often defined as 'sleep with a trace of awareness' and can be seen as an altered state of consciousness. On a separate note, if you suffer from insomnia, developing a yoga nidra practice may be of help. Anecdotally, people I have shared yoga nidra with in class and workshop settings have fed back to me that they experience much better sleep on the days when they have practised yoga nidra. This has been my personal experience too.

Yoga nidra is usually practised lying down and restorative yoga postures are ideal, because with yoga nidra it is important for the body to be in a position so comfortable that there is no desire to move. Poses such as Supported restorative savasana and Side-lying relaxation are just two examples that allow the physical body to be fully supported and encourage the release of muscular tension.

I would highly recommend experiencing yoga nidra live in a class or workshop setting if that is at all possible for you. Otherwise, recordings can be helpful as they allow you to more easily choose when you practise. I would suggest finding one particular recording that you like. That way, you are more likely to regularly practise it and by using the same recording it will be easier to become more familiar with the process and eventually be able to guide yourself. The experience of guiding yourself can take your experience of yoga nidra to an even deeper level (see p. 176 for yoga nidra teachers; recordings are also available on my website ucanyoga.co.uk).

The 61 points

A wonderful practice in its own right and a good way into yoga nidra is via the 61 points. This activates our vital energy centres (marma points and chakras) and is known for promoting deep rest and calm in both body and mind. (In Ayurvedic terms, marma points are energy points in the body, known in ancient Vedic times as bindu.) The 61 points is also known as shavayatra – inner pilgrimage through the body – and I came to learn of it as a practice from the Himalayan tradition as taught by Swami Rama. The 61 points often forms a part of guided yoga nidra practices, as a way to facilitate entering the state of yoga nidra. Therefore, as with nidra, the aim is not to fall asleep during the 61 points. Also, over time, this practice can, in fact, enhance your ability to concentrate – an incredibly valuable thing given the number of daily distractions coupled with the shortening attention spans so many of us increasingly experience.

Deeply relaxing and rejuvenating, the 61 points is usually practised in savasana. However, if lying down doesn't feel comfortable or safe for you then allow yourself to be fully supported in seated position for your practice. It involves guiding your focus systematically to each point around the body. For instance, this could be consciously placing your awareness on each point or visualising a point of light travelling to each point around the body. As with yoga nidra, there are many recordings of guided 61 points practices available (see below for a sample practice). Ideally, you will eventually guide yourself. In order to be able to self-guide, you will need to learn the points:

1 Eyebrow centre	13 Right shoulder joint	27 Centre of chest
2 Throat centre	14 Throat centre	(heart centre)
3 Right shoulder joint	15 Left shoulder joint	28 Middle of right chest
4 Right elbow joint	16 Left elbow joint	29 Centre of chest
5 Right wrist joint	17 Left wrist joint	30 Middle of left chest
6 Tip of right thumb	18 Tip of left thumb	31 Centre of chest
7 Tip of right index finger	19 Tip of left index finger	(end of 31 points)
8 Tip of right middle finger	20 Tip of left middle finger	32 Navel centre
9 Tip of right ring finger	21 Tip of left ring finger	33 Pelvic centre
10 Tip of right little finger	22 Tip of left little finger	34 Right hip joint
11 Right wrist joint	23 Left wrist joint	35 Right knee joint
12 Right elbow joint	24 Left elbow joint	36 Right ankle joint
	25 Left shoulder joint	37 Tip of right big toe
	26 Throat centre	38 Tip of second right toe

39 Tip of third right toe
40 Tip of fourth right toe
41 Tip of little toe
42 Right ankle joint
43 Right knee joint
44 Right hip joint
45 Pelvic centre
46 Left hip joint
47 Left knee joint
48 Left ankle joint
49 Tip of left big toe
50 Tip of second left toe
51 Tip of left third toe

52 Tip of left fourth toe
53 Tip of left little toe
54 Left ankle joint
55 Left knee joint
56 Left hip joint

57 Pelvic centre
58 Navel centre
59 Centre of chest
60 Throat centre
61 Eyebrow centre

That said, if this practice is brand new to you, it is advisable to begin with the 31 points and then when you're able to remain aware throughout (not fall asleep or lose your place during the sequence) you can move to the 61 points. To help you get started here is a 31 points and a 61 points practice you can try.

31 points guided practice

Set yourself up in a comfortable position and guide your awareness to your breathing. Notice the rise and fall of your breath. Guide your awareness to your navel. You might become aware of the gentle rise and fall of your belly as your body breathes. As you watch the breath, allow it to gradually smooth out until your inhale is approximately the same length as your exhale.

You will now bring your awareness to different points of the body, one by one. As you visit each point, the physical body becomes more relaxed.

Gently guide your awareness to the space between your eyebrows – your eyebrow centre, throat centre, tip of the right shoulder, right elbow, right wrist, tip of the right-hand thumb, index finger, middle finger, ring finger and little finger, right wrist, right elbow, tip of the right shoulder and back to the throat centre.

Tip of the left shoulder, left elbow, left wrist, tip of the left-hand thumb, index finger, middle finger, ring finger and little finger, left wrist, left elbow, tip of the left shoulder and back to the throat centre.

To the centre of the chest – the energetic heart centre, right side of the chest, centre of the chest, left side of the chest, centre of the chest. Allow the mind to rest here at the centre of the chest. Stay here resting with your awareness at heart centre for as long as you wish.

When you are ready to close your practice, slowly bring some gentle movement back to your body before guiding yourself carefully up to sitting or standing.

61 points guided practice

Allow yourself to make any adjustments you need to, ensuring that you're as comfortable as possible.

Bring your awareness to your breathing. Allow your breath to be even, with your inhale the same length as your exhale.

Guide your awareness to your eyebrow centre. At the eyebrow centre, visualise a soft and soothing point of light.

Now see that light move to the throat centre. And the tip of the right shoulder, right elbow and right wrist, tip of the right-hand thumb, right index finger, middle finger, ring finger and little finger, right wrist, right elbow, right shoulder and back to the throat centre – see that soothing point of light shining there.

Now see that light moving to the tip of the left shoulder, left elbow, left wrist, tip of the left-hand thumb, left index finger, middle finger, ring finger and little finger, left wrist, left elbow, tip of the left shoulder and back to the throat centre – point of light shining there, radiating.

To the centre of the chest. See that light shining at the centre of the chest, radiating to the right side of the chest, centre of the chest, left side of the chest, centre of the chest, the navel, the pelvic centre and to the right hip. See that soothing point of light shining at the right hip, right knee, right ankle, tip of the right big toe, second toe, third toe, fourth toe and little toe, right ankle, right knee, right hip and back to the pelvic centre.

Moving over to the left hip. See that soothing point of light shining at the left hip, left knee, left ankle, tip of the left big toe, second toe, third toe, fourth toe and little toe, left ankle, left knee, left hip and back to the pelvic centre.

Moving up to the navel. See that soothing point of light shining at the navel. Now see that light shining at the centre of the chest and at the throat centre, and up to the eyebrow centre. See that soothing light shining at the eyebrow centre. Rest in the light of your awareness at the eyebrow centre for as long as you wish.

When you're ready to close your practice, slowly bring some gentle movement back to your body before guiding yourself carefully up to sitting or standing.

May I be well – loving-kindness

What is loving-kindness, also known as metta bhavana? 'Metta' means 'non-romantic love', 'friendliness' and 'kindness', while 'bhavana' means 'cultivation' or 'development'. It comes from the Pali language and it is a practice from the Buddhist tradition for developing compassion. However, you don't have to be Buddhist to practise loving-kindness. It is a beautiful reminder that we are all connected and that you as well as others are worthy of tenderness and care.

So many of us find it hard to show ourselves the same compassion that we willingly show others. Loving-kindness can be a way to begin to redress that balance. Research has shown that loving-kindness can have numerous benefits, including subduing self-criticism and improving self-compassion, increasing vagal tone and the experience of more positive emotions, and it may even reduce chronic pain and decrease migraines. A 2008 study showed that even just a single short loving-kindness practice (less than 10 minutes) increased positive feelings towards strangers and feelings of social connection.

If you would like to give this a try for yourself, here is a loving-kindness meditation you can follow. The stages of this practice usually last for around five minutes:

Loving-kindness meditation

To begin your meditation, find a comfortable place to lie down or sit. Your eyes can be open or closed.

Start by offering loving-kindness to yourself by silently reciting several times:

'May I be well, may I be happy, may I be safe, may I live with ease.'

It's perfectly normal for the mind to wander, for distractions to arise, for thoughts to pop up. When this happens, just guide yourself back to reciting:

'May I be well, may I be happy, may I be safe, may I live with ease.'

Now think of a family member or friend – someone close to you. See them in your mind's eye as clearly as you can. Offer them what you have just offered yourself by silently reciting several times:

'May you be well, may you be happy, may you be safe, may you live with ease.'

Now, think of somebody who you know is having a difficult time and with this person in mind, continue to recite, again several times:

'May you be well, may you be happy, may you be safe, may you live with ease.'

Next, think of somebody you feel neutral about, someone you neither particularly like or dislike, and wish them well by silently reciting several times:

'May you be well, may you be happy, may you be safe, may you live with ease.'

Now, bringing to mind a person you do not like, offer loving-kindness to this person:

'May you be well, may you be happy, may you be safe, may you live with ease.'

If it feels too hard to do the latter, then return to offering loving-kindness to yourself by silently reciting:

'May I be well, may I be happy, may I be safe, may I live with ease.'

Complete your meditation by thinking of all these people, yourself included, and then extend your offering of loving-kindness to everyone around you, to everyone far away, to all beings everywhere, by silently reciting, several times:

'May all beings be well, may all beings be happy, may all beings be safe, may all beings live with ease.'

Starting the day on the right foot

It's so easy to slide into the day on autopilot and before you know it you're in a bad mood or flustered or overwhelmed and you're not even sure you know why. But it doesn't have to be that way.

We all have different lives and different schedules. This is not at all about formulating a perfect morning routine, like celebrities who are up for a daily 4 a.m. workout followed by a green smoothie (not that I have anything against green smoothies – in fact, I rather like them!). This is about finding small ways to help your mind and body into a more positive and intentional start to your day. Have a look at the suggestions that follow and pick what most resonates with you. It might be one thing or it might be three. Or maybe reading this creates inspiration for something totally different that you would like to do. It could be reading some inspirational words, it could be prayer. There is no one right way – what feels right for you is most important here.

Whatever you choose to do, your challenge – if you are willing to accept it – is to allow *at least the first 15 minutes of your day to be phone-free.* Let those first few minutes of your morning be a space in which you nurture yourself (hint: that does not mean hitting the snooze button). If the very idea of this seems selfish or fanciful, particularly if you have caring responsibilities, then this is a good place to remind yourself that you cannot give the best of yourself to others if you do not care for yourself first. It's the old oxygen mask analogy – you put your own mask on before helping others. Creating these pockets of time for you, whether for one minute or one hour, is an important way of honouring yourself.

Rather than reaching for your phone as soon as you open your eyes, here are some suggestions for starting your day that your nervous system will thank you for. Let's start your day on the right foot instead of the wrong one.

Before you get out of bed

Before you even get out of bed ask yourself this question: *How would I like to feel today?* Your answer could be a phrase, but really it only needs to be one word. If you like, place a hand on your heart and connect to your breath as you contemplate this. This need not take more than a minute or so – there's no need to overthink it.

Those moments just after you wake up, when you're semi-conscious, are a precious and ideal time to let your intuition guide you. This one word can be your intention for the day ahead. At various points through your day, reminding yourself of this word can help to bring you back to the present and to your intention. Plus doing so can provide the opportunity to make choices about your actions based on your intention.

From my own experience, this semi-conscious state is one of the best times for jotting down unfiltered thoughts and ideas, so if journaling appeals to you and you would like to take this a step further, here are a few questions for you to consider and free-write on (you can of course do this when you get out of bed if you prefer):

- What would your day look like and feel like if you took care of yourself first?
- What matters to you most?
- How can you do more of what matters today/this week?

Five minutes of breathing when you wake up

This is also something you can do while you're still in bed. Did you have a favourite pranayama practice (*see* pp. 126–8)? For example, psychic alternate nostril breathing is wonderful to do in the morning (as well as at the end of the day to help clear mental clutter). Also, this particular practice can help bring awareness to which of your nostrils feels more active when you wake up.

Morning bed yoga

How often do you wake up with a feeling of stiffness in your body and find yourself creaking your way out of bed? Here is a sequence involving gentle movements and stretches you can do to help loosen up and you don't even need to get out of bed to do it. If you can't/don't want to/don't have time to do the whole sequence, give yourself permission to do just one or two of these poses:

Full body stretch: Begin by pointing and flexing your feet, and stretching the arms and spreading the fingers.

Knees to chest: Follow this by hugging both knees in towards your chest. Either hold still here for a few breaths or gently rock from side to side.

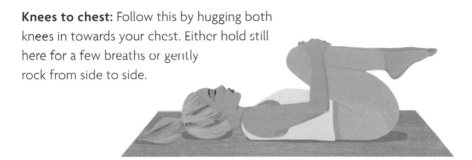

Knee circles: Rest your hands on your shins just below your knees or on the backs of your thighs. Begin to draw circles with your knees, moving your legs out, away from each other and then back together in the middle. After a few rotations, change the directions of your circles.

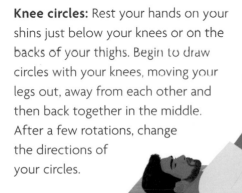

Windscreen wiper twists: Rest the soles of your feet on your bed. Toe-heel your feet apart so that your feet and knees are wider than hip-width. Take your arms out by your sides (your arms can be straight if you have room to stretch out or bend your elbows into a cactus shape). Allowing your breath and movements to be nice and steady, as you exhale, allow both knees to fall over to your right. Then as you inhale, bring both knees back to the middle where you started. Exhale as both knees fall over to the left. Continue with your Windscreen wiper twists, repeating a few times on each side, linking your breath to your movement.

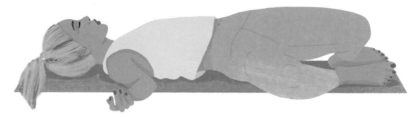

Hamstring stretch into Eye of the needle: Starting with the soles of both feet on your bed, hug your right knee in towards your chest and circle your right ankle one way and then the other. Extend your right foot up towards the ceiling and hold on to the back of your leg. Allow your right leg to be as straight as is comfortable. As you exhale, let your right heel reach towards the ceiling a little more. Hold here for two to five breaths.

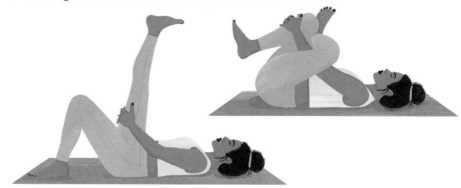

To move into Eye of the needle pose, rest your right thigh to the top of your left knee. This is step 1. You can choose to stay here or you can lift your left foot, thread your right arm through the middle of your legs and interlace your fingers on your left leg. This is step 2. As you exhale, hug your left thigh in towards you as far as feels comfortable. If you're staying at step 1, you have the option to rest your right palm on your right thigh and gently press your right thigh forward. Hold here for two to five breaths. Repeat your Hamstring stretch into Eye of the needle on your left leg.

Cat cow flow: Carefully roll over to one side and then come to an all-fours position. Allowing your movements to be steady and controlled, as you exhale, round your back into Cat pose, allowing your head to drop. As you inhale, allow your navel to drop towards your bed and your shoulders away from your ears into Cow pose. Continue with your Cat cow flow for several breaths.

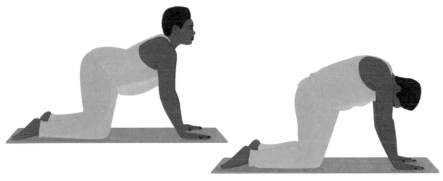

Hip circles: From your all-fours position, move your hips over to the right, back and down towards your right heel, over to your left heel, and continue all the way around to the left until you reach where you started. Continue your circles around to the right a few more times, allowing your elbows to bend as much as they need to in your circles. When you're ready to change direction, circle your hips around to the left.

When you are ready to bring your practice to a close, guide yourself to a comfortable kneeling or sitting position and pause here for a few breaths before moving on to your day.

After you get out of bed

Drinking warm water in the morning was something my mother introduced me to. Along with many habits I thought of as odd as a child and begrudgingly took up, it turns out that Mum really did know best! According to neuroscientist and author Dr Lisa Mosconi, warm water is more hydrating than cold and therefore vasodilating (promoting increased blood flow by expanding the blood vessels). This is also an Ayurvedic practice (where it is believed that drinking hot water is one of the best ways to detoxify). Adding lemon means added vitamin C.

If during the day you find that you are experiencing brain fog, fatigue, dizziness or having difficulty concentrating, note whether you have drunk any water. As obvious as it sounds to say 'stay hydrated', our brains are 80 per cent water and it takes as little as a 2 per cent to 4 per cent loss of water in the brain to bring on those symptoms.

Revisit your to-do list

If you have a to-do list from the night before (*see Putting the day to bed* on pp. 169–172), before your day fully kicks off can be a good time to revisit your list and see what you can cross off. Yes, really. Scrutinise each thing and see what actually does not need to be done today, what can be delegated or what isn't actually that important. If you're prone to over-estimating what you can do in a day, know that you are not alone.

Let the light In

Exposure to sunlight in the morning can help to increase serotonin and lower melatonin, helping to get you out of a sluggish state after waking up. Serotonin is a neurotransmitter known as one of our 'happy hormones' and it's thought to play a key role in regulating mood (low serotonin levels are associated with depression). We need melatonin for good sleep, but when we want to get up in the morning, not so much. However, serotonin gets converted to melatonin over the course of the day, so exposing ourselves to daylight in the morning can increase the production of serotonin and has a positive knock-on effect on our sleep that night.

Admittedly, the amount of bright sunlight we get will depend on where we live and the time of year. Nevertheless, draw back those curtains or blinds when you get out of bed and take the opportunity to get outside in the morning if you're able to. Maybe it could be a walk as part of your journey to work or taking your children to school. Maybe it's going for a run. Or if you're fortunate enough to have outdoor space at home, then it could be sitting outside for a while (with your warm water or breakfast or re-visiting your to-do list) if your schedule allows.

Moving through your day

'Boundaries' has become a buzzword. However, it's not necessarily clear why setting and holding boundaries is important – and what is a boundary anyway? A personal boundary is a limit on what you will and will not accept based on compassion and kindness towards yourself. From a yoga perspective, if you consider ahimsa, the first of the yamas, which is the first of the eight limbs of yoga (see p. 19), it means non-harming and it's important to remember that non-harming includes you too, so setting healthy personal boundaries as well as respecting the boundaries of others is a way of practising ahimsa.

Setting your personal boundaries

Despite the implications of the word 'boundary', having personal boundaries is not about cutting yourself off from others. If anything, it's the opposite. Healthy, compassionate personal boundaries can, among other things:

- allow for the relationships in your life to become richer and deeper
- make life happier
- bring peace
- protect your mental health
- improve self-esteem
- open up space to do more of what matters to you
- allow you to give to others from a place of generosity and fullness

When you don't have healthy personal boundaries, it can lead to:

- depletion
- resentment
- feeling taken advantage of
- imbalanced and damaged relationships

- self-abandonment
- impaired mental health
- burnout

Some of the above can also be what it feels like when a boundary is crossed. Looking at this list of what not having boundaries can feel like may be of help in working out your own boundaries. A few other suggestions for boundary setting include:

- Get clear on what you are willing (and not willing) to accept and why. If you get stuck here, ask yourself: What would be the consequences for me of accepting what I know that deep down I should not?
- Work out how to articulate this so that you are able to communicate your boundary to to others when and if necessary (e.g. if a boundary is crossed).
- Know that your boundaries can vary and be flexible depending on the situation and relationship

For instance, do you feel really drained after spending a lot of time with certain people or resentful after having agreed to do something? These are examples of situations that would benefit from examination in order to amend your behaviour and set a clearer boundary for your well-being.

This can be difficult if you are a people-pleaser. However, for your own sake you need to do this. Give yourself grace and know that it will take practice. Sometimes this will mean disappointing other people, which may be a challenge if they have been used to you always saying 'Yes'. In these instances, what may be required is gradually amending your behaviour so that those people know that you will not say 'Yes' all the time. What I have found is that the people who truly care about you will respect your wishes.

If you think that you don't deserve this for yourself, then it's worth going back a few steps and asking why you feel this way. You are allowed to change. Just because things have always been a certain way and that's what everyone has been used to, it doesn't mean it has to stay that way. If you're looking for external permission, then I am giving you that permission here and now, and letting you know that you absolutely do deserve to protect your peace.

Honouring your threshold

We are all different and therefore we all have different thresholds when it comes to how much we can handle, whether that's workload, responsibilities, how many people we feel comfortable being around at any one time, what we can actually do based our energy levels at the time... the list can be endless. Whatever your threshold is related to, it may change over time or depending on the situation and in a way honouring your threshold can be related to your personal boundaries.

Trying to push beyond what you know is a limit for you, or feeling as though you are being forced to do so, is very likely to cause you suffering in some way. It is important to take an honest look at what you can control in order to look after your own well-being. This will look different for each of us, but a few examples could include:

- not overscheduling yourself
- getting into the practice of taking things off your to do list (see *Starting the day on the right foot* on pp. 155–9)
- practising holding and communicating your boundaries where necessary
- get into the practice of saying yes only when you really want to
- remembering the phrase 'Let me get back to you' when you need time to think about a request (caveat: if you already know the answer is no, it is fairer on you and everyone around you to say so upfront)

Mono-tasking over multi-tasking

Multi-tasking is overrated and stressful. If productivity and peace is your goal, then mono-tasking – working on one thing at a time rather than several – is the way forward.

For decades, multi-tasking was lauded and encouraged as it was seen as a way of being efficient. In more recent years, research has shown this to be

FOR ME, BOUNDARIES ARE PERSONAL

When someone, a Black woman I respect, told me that she saw me as a 'boundaried person', I took that as a compliment. I also took it as a sign of progress.

My name is Paula and I am a people-pleaser in recovery. I also happen to be a Black woman. These things are relevant and inextricably linked when it comes to boundaries.

Something I have found throughout my life, and something that perplexed me for a long time, was the level of anger or punishment I faced for simply saying the word 'No'. At the very least, the response to my 'No' would be dismissal and a dogged persistence to try and grind me down until I said 'Yes'. If you're someone who does not identify as Black, who is reading this and thinking 'Yes, but' or 'I experience this too', please do consider that we all live at different intersections and that I am talking about a specific lived experience that not only I, but many Black women especially, will understand on a deep level. I am talking about 'the angry Black woman' stereotype.

It took me years to realise that my people-pleasing was tied to trying to avoid or deflect the anger and the bullying I would be subjected to ▶

false. Multi-tasking may seduce us into thinking we are succeeding at doing everything, but in reality it's not possible to give our full attention to and process lots of things at once. The chances are that those things are not being done as well as they could be, plus mistakes are more likely, and if there could be consequences to such mistakes is multi-tasking really worth it? A 2016 study found that as little as a two- or three-second interruption of a task to switch to another can double mistakes while a 2009 study showed that heavy multi-taskers were less able to focus, less productive and less able to remember information compared to people doing one thing at a time.

So not only could mono-tasking save you time, it is less stressful for your brain. Here are a few suggestions to help you let go of multi-tasking and make mono-tasking a habit:

and, to be frank, to try and have an easier life, because on the other side of it was (and still is) being perceived as 'angry' or 'difficult' for saying 'No', despite having not raised my voice or expressed anger at any point. Being labelled as 'the angry Black woman' can have dire consequences and so, for a long time, this fear prevented me from having and holding reasonable boundaries.

In order to change, it took getting older, realising that the people who really cared about me would understand and respect me, and, most importantly, that looking after myself mattered.

Boundaries matter because looking after yourself matters. Looking after yourself matters because you matter.

I feel it is important to write about this here in the context of my personal experience, because it is essential to understand that part of setting our own boundaries is respecting the boundaries of others. That includes being able to accept someone else's 'No'. Just as others are not automatically entitled to your energy, your time or your resources, you are not entitled to theirs. And if you find that you do feel entitled, be willing to interrogate why this might be so. Care and consideration for self is not divorced from care and consideration for others.

Reduce distractions: Whether it's pinging noises from your phone or the lure of social media, not only do distractions take your mind away from the task you're working on, they can make it harder to regain your focus to pick up where you left off. If, for instance, you know that you are prone to browsing online, consider using an app and/or site-blocking software for the duration of the time that you want to focus on your task, so that the temptation is eliminated.

Divide your day into chunks: Look at your to-do list for the day and think about what is most pressing. Big things that you know cannot be done in one go can be broken down further. It can also be very helpful to have an understanding of your own rhythms. When in the day do you feel more alert? When in the day does your energy dip? That way you can more easily work out when is best for you to schedule things that require deep concentration versus things that do not.

Allocate time to each task: For example, if I am working on an intensive task (especially if it involves sitting at a computer), I find that working in 30-minute bursts followed by a break of about five minutes really helps me to focus, and is much more enjoyable and effective than pressing on with gritted teeth and no respite until a task feels done. Experiment to see what works best for you based on your own rhythms and your particular situation. Sometimes external circumstances mean that doing this is challenging, so focus on what you are able to control.

Smart use of your smartphone

I am old enough to remember life before mobile phones. I didn't grow up with them and didn't get my first mobile phone until after university. At that point, mobile phones were just for calls and texts. In a relatively short space of time after that, technology advanced and the smartphone was born. I did not really see what all the fuss was about, but then I got my first smartphone and within days I was hooked. I tell this story about my own experience to say that it is not only people who grew up with this technology that can be quickly drawn in.

There are many benefits to smartphones. They help us stay connected to family and friends, they capture memories, provide entertainment and they can help make aspects of our day-to-day lives easier. One of the benefits of mobile phones is that they give us the ability to be always in contact. That's also one of the biggest downsides, as it comes with the sense that others may expect us to always be available, coupled with the expectation of instant responses to messages. This doesn't mean that you need to give up your smartphone (unless of course you want to). Instead, you can lean in to being more mindful in how you choose to use it.

Let downtime work for you

If you have a smartphone with a downtime function, then using it can be a great gift to yourself. It can free up time and headspace, as well as helping you to wind down at the end of the day as you will be exposing yourself to less blue light (*see Putting the day to bed* on pp. 169–72). When I started using downtime regularly, it clearly revealed how much time I had been wasting on my phone, particularly on social media. Speaking of which ...

Social media use

If you do use social media, it's very likely that you have found yourself spending more time than you intended scrolling through your feeds. It's so easy to do, and so easy to feel guilty about, and if this is your experience you are far from alone. The trouble is, social media is designed to be addictive and to keep you scrolling. But if you do not want to give up social media, there are ways you can use it more consciously rather than feeling as though it is using you. Having a cut-off (for example, not going on to social media after 8 p.m.), deleting apps from your phone and accessing them only via a desktop, or deciding to have social media breaks can all be incredibly helpful. Personally, I have found that the latter has worked best and most consistently. For me, it started with a week-long social media break and from that Switch Off Sundays were born.

Switch Off Sundays

Back in 2017 I realised that my social media scrolling was becoming a problem. I regularly found myself on the apps on my phone late at night and then reaching for my phone as soon as I woke up in the morning. What had started as a few minutes a day became the thing I reached for when there seemed to be gaps or transitions in my day – travelling on the train to teach a class, sitting on the bus in traffic, waiting in cafés between classes. This was a stage when I went to different parts of the city most days for work. At first looking at social media felt like it gave me a boost, but after a while I found that I didn't feel good after spending time on those apps – and it was a lot of time, as my weekly phone report told me.

Aside from studies showing that the blue light emitted from our screens can hinder sleep, research also suggests a link between spending extended time on social media and experiencing negative mental health outcomes. With mental health in mind, it is also worth remembering that you always have the choice to unfollow and block on social media too.

I decided to take a week off social media and to my surprise it was nowhere near as difficult as I imagined it would be. In fact, I felt better quite quickly. A few outcomes from just a week away from social media included:

* more time!
* a brighter mood
* better sleep
* the space for more creative ideas to come through
* enjoying reading again (real books rather than via an electronic device)

I have taken more weeks off social media since, but one thing I began straight after that week was making my Sundays a social media-free zone. It means that I can still enjoy the positive aspects of social media without it taking up too much of my time. An interesting side-effect of Switch Off Sundays is that they have gradually and naturally reduced the amount of time I spend on social media over the course of the whole week. If you are looking to spend a little less time online, then how about joining me for Switch Off Sundays? This can be an ideal place to start if a week or more feels like too much of a leap for you at the moment. Also, that one day a week adds up to 52 days over the course of the year. Just think what else you could be doing – in real life – with that time.

Emails

Related to the above, if emails tend to form a large part of your day, rather than reading and responding as soon as an email arrives, consider whether selecting certain points in the day to check in and respond to emails may work better. Depending on your work or life situation, this may be a more effective use of your time. It might look like dedicating specific chunks of time to dealing with emails two to three times per day, such as in the morning, after lunch and then once more at the end of the day. Also, for the times in between, consider whether having an automated email response, communicating to email senders that you will be looking at and responding to emails at specific times, might be helpful. This can help to manage the expectations of others and reduce any pressure you may otherwise feel to respond instantly (*see Allocate time to each task* on p. 166).

Putting the day to bed

As with *Starting the day on the right foot* (*see* pp. 157–9), this is not about formulating an exacting routine that must be stuck to day in, day out. Begin with one thing. It doesn't need to be overwhelming. What truly works for you is more likely to become habit.

Here are a few suggestions for winding down well and setting yourself up for restful sleep. Feel free to take what resonates and put aside the rest.

Your last meal (and drink) of the day

Have you always had your dinner at a certain time, but now find when you go to bed that you still have a feeling of food 'sitting' in your stomach? If so, then it's worth looking at whether it's possible to have your last meal of the day at an earlier time. Eating too close to bedtime can disrupt sleep at any stage of our lives, though it is also worth noting that there may be a reason why what has worked for you in the past doesn't work for you now. If you feel aware that this is having a negative impact on your sleep, but your schedule doesn't allow you to eat dinner earlier, then maybe it's possible to have your largest meal earlier in the day and let your evening meal be lighter.

On a related note, if you've been experiencing trouble sleeping here are a few things to consider in relation to food and drink consumption:

Do you regularly consume caffeine? For instance, the caffeine in tea usually leaves your system four to six hours *after* you drink it. Also, you could be consuming caffeine via things like fizzy drinks or chocolate, especially chocolate with a high cocoa content, or even your cup of hot cocoa right before bedtime. Speaking from my own experience, it took me a while to work out that my habit of having a couple of squares of dark chocolate after my evening meal was having a negative impact on my sleep.

Do you drink alcohol? As alcohol is mostly sugar, a sugar spike resulting from your liver breaking it down means that drinking in the evenings, especially close to bedtime, can disturb your sleep and for some people may also bring on night sweats. Speaking of night sweats ...

Could spicy foods be a culprit? If you're in a stage of menopause (perimenopausal, menopausal or postmenopausal), it is worth knowing that spicy foods can bring on night sweats and hot flushes. Hot drinks too close to bedtime may have a similar effect.

None of this is to suggest giving up things that you like or being rigid – it is more about developing an awareness of any habits that may inadvertently be having a negative impact on the quality of your sleep and rest. It means you can discover what works best for you and amend things accordingly, most of the time. It also means that if you do choose to have a glass of red wine in the evening while catching up with a friend, you're doing so from a place of knowledge. In my case, I still eat dark chocolate (a non-negotiable for me!), I just have it earlier in the day.

Turn the lights down low (after sunset)

Exposure to light such as sunlight at the right time can be helpful for boosting our alertness. However, boosting our alertness is not going to help us put the day to bed. Research has shown that blue light – in this case, the light from screens – can suppress melatonin levels. It is now common knowledge that looking at screens too close to bedtime can disrupt sleep for this reason. To reduce your exposure to blue light in the evenings, as well as using the downtime facility on your smartphone if you have one, you could also introduce a screen-time cut-off for, say, two hours before bedtime. Maybe this means listening to music or reading – not on a screen – instead of an evening box-set marathon on the TV.

On a related note, very bright artificial lighting can impact melatonin and therefore your ability to get to sleep too. If it's within your power to adjust the lighting in your home, then you could try low lighting after the sun goes down. Aside from signalling to your brain that it is time to wind down, lower lighting can also create a feeling of cosiness. Try going for lamps and lower-wattage bulbs rather than strong overhead lights. If you like candles, this could be a perfect way of enjoying them. There is another way you can use your candles too.

Candle-gazing to calm the mind

'Tratakam' means 'gaze' or 'look' and candle-gazing is a way of practising tratakam (the technique of gazing at an object). This also relates to dharana (focused concentration), the sixth of the eight limbs of yoga (see p. 19). As well as calming the mind, aiding sleep is said to be one of the other benefits of this practice. Here is a candle-gazing meditation for you to try:

Light a candle and place it on a flat surface approximately one to one and a half metres in front of you.

Sit in a comfortable position with the candle in your eyeline, in a position where you won't strain your neck if you look at the flame.

Close your eyes and guide your awareness to your breathing. Allow your breath to be smooth and steady.

After several breaths, open your eyes. With a soft gaze, look at the candle flame. Guide your awareness to the brightest part of the flame for approximately 10 to 15 seconds.

Close your eyes again and see whether you're able to visualise the flame. Do not worry if you're not able to visualise it – the aim is not to strive. If you can visualise the flame with closed eyes, hold the image softly to avoid creating any tension.

When the visualisation of the flame fades, or after 10 to 15 seconds (whichever is longer), open your eyes again and repeat the above process – softly gazing at the candle flame, then closing your eyes to visualise the flame – three times.

When you're ready to close your candle-gazing practice, guide your awareness back to the rise and fall of your breathing for five to eight breaths.

Over time, with regular practice, you may wish to gradually increase the duration of gazing at the flame (up to one minute) and visualising the flame behind closed eyes (up to four minutes).

Nightly notes

If you are prone to rumination or find that your mind is full then one tip that can be helpful is to take a notebook or piece of paper and 'brain dump' – get all the stuff that's bothering you in your head out on to the page. If you know Julia Cameron's The Artist's Way, you will be familiar with 'morning pages'. I call this 'bedtime pages', because before I go to bed I like to free-write, with a pen and paper, just letting my hand write without censoring myself, until I fill at least one whole page or it feels right to stop. Sometimes,

I then rip that piece of paper up and throw it away as a further symbol of letting all that negative stuff go before I go to sleep. If this appeals to you then do give it a try — it can be surprisingly cathartic. It is a good idea to have a notebook and pen that live next to your bed so that you always have the option to do bedtime pages if you choose.

Plan for tomorrow

If to-do lists are your thing, the evening is a good time to write your list for the next day. Not only does this save you time in the morning, but much like the bedtime pages, it means that your tasks for the next day are less likely to be whirling around in your head while you're lying in bed trying to go to sleep. In addition, having your list ready and waiting means you can review (and, ideally, reduce) it in the morning, as suggested in *After you get out of bed* (*see* p. 160).

Breathing before bedtime

Bee breath is just one of the breathing practices that may be helpful at bedtime. Left nostril breathing (chandra bhedana) is another wonderful practice to calm the mind (*see* pp. 131–4 for full instructions on how to practise both).

Bedtime body scan

Instead of counting sheep, try a bedtime body scan once you've got into bed (*see* pp. 146–8 for guidance). It's a good idea to learn your preferred sequence by heart so that you can guide yourself and not need to rely on a recording played through your smartphone or other device (if in doubt, start with the shorter body scan systematic relaxation). Don't worry about learning it word for word. Rather, think about becoming familiar with the specific points and the process — for example, working from the head down or from the toes up. If you like, you could start with the *Tense and release* exercise (*see* pp. 30–31) beforehand to help with letting go of muscular tension.

Going forward – not the end, but the beginning

I hope the contents of this book have provided you with some practices and inspiration for looking after yourself well. You deserve to treat yourself just as you would a precious loved one. We live in a world that often doesn't want us to rest – there will always be things to do, demands on our time or distractions begging for our attention – so it's up to you to claim it. Knock busyness off its pedestal and place rest there in its rightful place. Hustle is overrated. Life is not just about ticking off accomplishments. Get still, rest and listen. Pause long enough to hear the voice of your inner wisdom, so that you can be clear about what truly matters to you – and then carve out space in your life for more of that.

Wishing you rest, calm and joy.

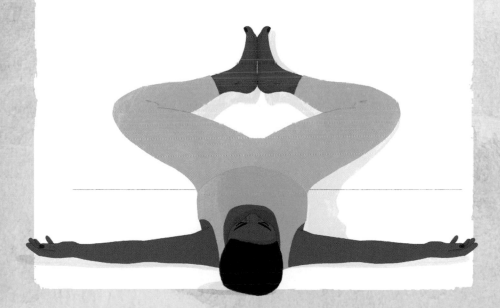

REFERENCES

Note: References are ordered by their appearance in the text, not alphabetically.

Part 1: Rest

Hammond, C. and Lewis, G. (2016) 'The Rest Test', BBC/Hubbub, ncbi.nlm.nih.gov/books/NBK453237/

Lee, H., Xie, L. et al. (2015) 'The Effect of Body Posture on Brain Glymphatic Transport', *JNeurosci* 5(31): 11034–11044

Tyagi, A. and Cohen, M. (2016) 'Yoga and heart rate variability', *Int J Yoga*, www.ncbi.nlm.nih.gov/pmc/articles/PMC4959333/

See also the work of Stephen Porges on Polyvagal Theory

Hartono, J.L., Mahadeva, S. and Goh, K.L. (2012) 'Anxiety and depression in various functional gastrointestinal disorders: Do differences exist?' *J Dig Dis* 13(5): 252–7.

Lee, C., Doo, E., Choi, J.M. et al. (2017) 'The increased level of depression and anxiety in irritable bowel syndrome patients compared with healthy controls', *J Neurogastroenterol Motil* 23(3): 349–362

Popa, S.L. and Dumitrascu, D.L. (2015) 'Anxiety and IBS revisited: Ten years later', *Clujul Med* 88(3): 253–257

Ankrom, S. (2021) 'Gastrointestinal symptoms and anxiety disorders', *Very Well Mind*, bit.ly/3tGQvJH.

Anxiety & Depression Association of America. 'Facts and Statistics'. www.adaa.org/understanding-anxiety/facts-statistics

Forbes, B. (2011) *Yoga for Emotional Balance* (Boulder, CO: Shambala)

Ekholm, B., Spulber, S. and Adler, M. (2020) 'A randomized controlled study of weighted chain blankets…', *JCSM* 16(9): 1567–1577

Champagne, T., Mullen, B., Krishnamurty, S., Dickson, D. and Gao, R. (2018) 'Controlled Study of Chain Blanket for Insomnia', https://bit.ly/3lqpcQ6

World Health Organization (2020) 'Depression', www.who.int/news-room/fact-sheets/detail/depression

James, S.L., Abate, D., Abate K.H. et al. (2018) 'Global, regional, and national incidence, prevalence, and years lived with disability …', *The Lancet* 392(10159): 1789–1858

Abi-Habib, R. and Patrick Luyten, P. (2013) 'The role of dependency and self-criticism in the relationship between anger and depression', *Personality and Individual Differences* 55(8): 921–925

NHS UK (2021) 'PMS', www.nhs.uk/conditions/pre-menstrual-syndrome/

Halme, J. et al. (1984) 'Retrograde menstruation in healthy women and in patients with endometriosis', *Obstet Gynecol* 64(2): 151–4

Bieber, E.J., Sanfilippo, J.S., Mahmood I., Shafi, I.R. & Shafi, M.L. (2015) *Clinical Gynecology* (Cambridge: Cambridge University Press)

Kerr, M.G. et al. (1964) 'Studies of the Inferior Vena Cava in Late Pregnancy', *British Medical Journal* 1(5382): 522–4, 532–533

Green, R. and Santoro N. (2009) 'Menopausal Symptoms and Ethnicity, the Study of Women's Health Across the Nation', *Womens Health* 5(2):127–33

Green, R. et al. (August 2010) 'Menopausal symptoms within a Hispanic cohort: SWAN', *Climacteric* 13(4):376–84

Arruda, M.S. et al. (2003) 'Time elapsed from onset of symptoms to diagnosis of endometriosis in a cohort study of Brazilian women', *Human Reproduction* 18:4 756–759

Kumar, A. et al. (May 2020) 'Effect of Yoga as Add-On Therapy in Migraine: A Randomized Clinical Trial', *Neurology* 94(21)

Part 2: Calm

Xiao Ma, X., Yue, Gong, Z.Q. et al. (2017) 'The Effect of Diaphragmatic Breathing on Attention, Negative Affect and Stress in Healthy Adults', *Front Psychol* 8: 874

Kaur, A. and Mitra, M. (2019) 'Effect of oropharyngeal exercises and Pranayama on snoring, daytime sleepiness and quality of sleep …', *European Respiratory Journal* 54: PA577

Jafari, H. et al. (2020) 'Can Slow Deep Breathing Reduce Pain? An Experimental Study Exploring Mechanisms', *J Pain* 21(9–10):1018–1030

Sharma V.K. et al. (2013) 'Effect of fast and slow pranayama on perceived stress and cardiovascular parameters in young health-care students', *IJOY*, 6:2 104–110

Pramanik, T. et al. (2010) 'Immediate effect of a slow pace breathing exercise Bhramari pranayama on blood pressure and heart rate', *Nepal Med Coll* 12(3):154–7

Floyd, K. (2014) 'Relational and Health Correlates of Affection Deprivation', *Western Journal of Communication* 78:4, 383–403

Gallace, A., Torta, D. et al. (2011) 'The analgesic effect of crossing the arms', *Pain* 152(6): 1418–23

Burel, R., Goodin, T. et al. (2015) 'Oxytocin – A Multifunctional Analgesic for Chronic Deep Tissue Pain', *Curr Pharm Des* 21(7): 906–913

Poerio, G.L. et al. (2018) 'More than a feeling: Autonomous sensory meridian response (ASMR) … Therapeutic benefits for physical and mental health', *PLoS One*, 13(6): e0196645

Chevalier, G., Patel S. et al. (2019) 'The Effects of Grounding (Earthing) on Bodyworkers' Pain and Overall Quality of Life: A Randomized Controlled Trial', *EXPLORE* 15(3): 181–190

Chevalier, G. (2015) 'The effect of grounding the human body on mood', *Psychol Rep* 116(2): 534–42

Bach, D., Groesbeck, G., Stapleton, P. et al. (2019) 'Clinical EFT (Emotional Freedom Techniques) Improves Multiple Physiological Markers of Health', *J Evid Based Integr Med* 24: 2515690X18823691

Ussher, M., Spatz, A., Copland, C. et al. (2014) 'Immediate effects of a brief mindfulness-based body scan on patients with chronic pain', *J Behav Med*, 37(1): 127–34

Hoge, Elizabeth A. et al. (2013) 'Randomized Controlled Trial of Mindfulness Meditation for Generalized Anxiety Disorder: Effects on Anxiety and Stress Reactivity', *J Clin Psychiatry* 74(8): 786–792

Shahar, B., Szsepsenwol, O., Zilcha-Mano, S. et al. (2015) 'A wait-list randomized controlled trial of loving-kindness meditation programme for self-criticism', *Clin Psychol Psychother* 22(4): 346–56.

Kok, B.E., Coffey, K.A., Cohn, M.A. et al. (2013) 'How positive emotions build physical health: perceived positive social connections account for the upward spiral between positive emotions and vagal tone', *Psychol Sci* 24(7): 1123–32

Carson, J.W., Keefe, F.J., Lynch, T.R. et al. (2005) 'Loving-kindness meditation for chronic low back pain: results from a pilot trial', *J Holist Nurs*, 23(3):287–304

Tonelli, M.E. and Wachholtz, A.B. (2014) 'Meditation-based treatment yielding immediate relief for meditation-naïve migraineurs', *Pain Manag Nurs* 15(1): 36–40.

Hutcherson, C.A., Seppala, E.M. and Gross, J.J. (2008) 'Loving-kindness meditation increases social connectedness', *Emotion* 8(5):720–4

Mark, G., Gudith, D. et al. (2008) 'The Cost of Interrupted Work: More Speed and Stress', *CHI '08: Proceedings of the SIGCHI Conference* 107–110

Gorlick, A. (2009) 'Media multitaskers pay mental price, Stanford study shows', news.stanford. edu/2009/08/24/multitask-research-study-082409/

Teachers

Uma Dinsmore-Tuli and Nirlipta Tuli: yoganidranetwork.org

Bo Forbes: boforbes.com

Judith Hanson Lasater: judithhansonlasater.com

Tracee Stanley: traceeyoga.com

Books

Cameron, Julia (2016) *The Artist's Way* (New York: Penguin)

Forbes, Bo (2011) *Yoga for Emotional Balance* (Boulder, CO: Shambala)

Hanson Lasater, Judith (2011) *Relax and Renew: Restful Yoga for Stressful Times* (Boulder, CO: Shambala)

Parker, Dr Gail (2020) *Restorative Yoga for Ethnic and Race-Based Stress and Trauma* (London: Singing Dragon)

Stanley, Tracee (2021) *Radiant Rest* (Boulder, CO: Shambala)

Resources

samaritans.org.
depressionuk.org
mind.org.uk
endometriosis.org